INTERPERSONAL PSYCHOTHERAPY *for* DEPRESSED OLDER ADULTS

INTERPERSONAL PSYCHOTHERAPY *for* DEPRESSED OLDER ADULTS

Gregory A. Hinrichsen *and*
Kathleen F. Clougherty

American Psychological Association • *Washington, DC*

Second Printing December, 2010
Published by
American Psychological Association
750 First Street, NE
Washington, DC 20002
www.apa.org

To order
APA Order Department
P.O. Box 92984
Washington, DC 20090-2984
Tel: (800) 374-2721; Direct: (202) 336-5510
Fax: (202) 336-5502; TDD/TTY: (202) 336-6123
Online: www.apa.org/books/
E-mail: order@apa.org

In the U.K., Europe, Africa, and the Middle East, copies may be ordered from
American Psychological Association
3 Henrietta Street
Covent Garden, London
WC2E 8LU England

Typeset in Goudy by Stephen D. McDougal, Mechanicsville, MD

Printer: Sheridan Books, Ann Arbor, MI
Cover Designer: Naylor Design, Washington, DC
Technical/Production Editor: Dan Brachtesende

The opinions and statements published are the responsibility of the authors, and such opinions and statements do not necessarily represent the policies of the American Psychological Association.

Library of Congress Cataloging-in-Publication Data

Hinrichsen, Gregory A., 1951-
    Interpersonal psychotherapy for depressed older adults / Gregory A. Hinrichsen and Kathleen F. Clougherty.
        p. cm.
    Includes bibliographical references and index.
    ISBN 1-59147-361-6
    1. Older people—Mental health. 2. Interpersonal psychotherapy. 3. Older people—Mental health services. 4. Depression, Mental. I. Clougherty, Kathleen F. II. Title.
[DNLM: 1. Depression—therapy—Aged. 2. Psychotherapy —methods—Aged.
3. Interpersonal Relations—Aged. WM 171 H664i 2006]

RC451.4.A5H558 2006
618.97'68527—dc22   2005024207

British Library Cataloguing-in-Publication Data
A CIP record is available from the British Library.

Printed in the United States of America
First Edition

For Rob—at the top of my interpersonal inventory.
—Gregory A. Hinrichsen

To my mentors, family, and friends: Thank you.
—Kathleen F. Clougherty

CONTENTS

Foreword . . . . *ix*

Preface . . . . *xi*

Acknowledgments . . . . *xv*

Chapter 1.　Gerontology: Exploring the Worlds of
Older Adults 3

Chapter 2.　Depression and Older Adults 21

Chapter 3.　Interpersonal Psychotherapy: Origins, Structure,
Research, and Applications 43

Chapter 4.　Interpersonal Psychotherapy for Late-Life
Depression 61

Chapter 5.　The Initial Sessions 75

Chapter 6.　Grief 93

Chapter 7.　Interpersonal Role Disputes 111

Chapter 8.　Role Transitions 133

Chapter 9.　Interpersonal Deficits 153

Chapter 10.　Termination 175

Chapter 11.　Issues in Implementation of Interpersonal
Psychotherapy With Older Adults 183

Chapter 12.   Next Steps   195

Resources   201

References..   205

Index..   221

About the Authors.....................................   227

FOREWORD

When interpersonal psychotherapy (IPT) was first invented by my late husband Gerald L. Klerman and myself, the conventional wisdom was that older patients could not benefit from psychotherapy. The model patient was a young, highly educated woman. This situation has changed dramatically. A recent analysis by Mark Olfson, MD,[1] on the usage and characteristics of patients in psychotherapy over the past decades revealed that about 3% of the population received some psychotherapy during a given year. This situation did not change between 1987 and 1997, when the data were collected. However, the nature of psychotherapy and the characteristics of the patients receiving it have changed dramatically. Psychotherapy has changed from long term to brief, and the age of those receiving psychotherapy has increased.

This book by Hinrichsen and Clougherty captures these trends. They describe a brief psychotherapy (IPT) that is evidence-based and adapted for older patients with depression. What is reassuring to read in their excellent clinical material is the seamless adaptation of IPT for an older population. As they note, IPT required no change. However, their book adds to the literature by providing a context for the problems that an older patient brings to psychotherapy. Concern about death, grief, medical illnesses, and long-term disputes becomes more salient as the patient ages. None of these problems are unique to older patients, but they do occur more frequently in this population. Hinrichsen and Clougherty have applied their skill and experience in using IPT to the problems of older patients. Their clinical material

[1]Olfson, M., Marcus, S. C., Druss, B., & Pincus, H. A. (2002). National trends in the use of outpatient psychotherapy. *American Journal of Psychiatry, 159,* 1914–1920.

alone is worth the price of this book. It is also heartening to see that the strategies of IPT can be so readily used in different patient groups.

Myrna M. Weissman, PhD
Professor of Epidemiology in Psychiatry
Chief, Division of Clinical and Genetic Epidemiology
College of Physicians and Surgeons of Columbia University

PREFACE

Increasing numbers of Americans are entering into later life. The size of the older population will double in the next 25 years, and in 2030 one fifth of the United States population will be 65 years of age or older. Given these facts, we suspect that most psychologists entering the field now will see older adults in clinical practice during their careers. We can remember a time when it was an empirical question whether psychotherapy could benefit older adults. Now a solid body of clinical research studies demonstrates that older adults benefit from psychotherapy as much as do younger adults. Most psychotherapies that were developed for younger adults can be used with older adults.

The field of psychology has placed increasing emphasis on the use of psychotherapies that have been demonstrated empirically to work. Although empirically supported treatments (ESTs) in psychology have their critics, ESTs are part of a broader movement for accountability in health care. Interpersonal psychotherapy (IPT) is one of several psychotherapeutic interventions that have demonstrated utility in the treatment of depression. Hinrichsen's initial interest in IPT was based on findings from research conducted at his home institution showing that interpersonally relevant factors longitudinally predicted clinical outcomes among a group of hospitalized older adults with major depression. By logical extension, interpersonal factors seemed important in treating late-life depression, and IPT explicitly targets those factors. Clougherty's interest in IPT similarly arose out of a research endeavor. As part of a research study of HIV-positive individuals with depression, she was trained to conduct IPT by one of its originators, Gerald Klerman.

Although the genesis of our interest in IPT was research, continued use of IPT in clinical practice has been fueled by other factors. We have found that IPT works in clinical practice: The majority of our clients with depression get better. IPT offers a framework for the treatment of depression and also considerable clinical latitude. IPT engages therapist and client in a practical and hopeful dialogue in an effort to decrease depressive symptoms and improve quality of life. After many years as psychotherapists, we found that learning IPT improved our clinical work with depressed clients and infused our work with clinical clarity and deeper professional satisfaction. We believe that even our colleagues who have been wary of ESTs will find IPT to be a clinically versatile tool that will build on the clinician's existing strengths. When conducting IPT workshops we are always pleased to hear participants remark that they currently use elements of IPT in their existing clinical work. We believe that these remarks reflect the fact that IPT was developed by experienced therapists who drew on their own clinical experience to identify which elements of their therapeutic work seemed most helpful to persons with depression.

Our own collaboration began in 1993. John Markowitz, MD, at New York Hospital–Cornell Medical Center and Clougherty had recently started an IPT training program in which Gregory Hinrichsen participated. Hinrichsen was supervised by Clougherty in his application of IPT to the treatment of late-life depression. Since that time, we have worked together in a variety of IPT-related projects, including IPT workshops at professional meetings.

This volume applies IPT, as developed by Gerald Klerman, Myrna Weissman, and their colleagues, to older adults with depression. It also draws on IPT research on late-life depression conducted by Ellen Frank, Charles Reynolds, and their collaborators at the University of Pittsburgh. With cognizance of broader issues that apply to psychotherapeutic work with older adults, the original IPT framework for the treatment of depression in younger adults can be applied to older adults. The fact that IPT can be applied so readily to older adults attests to the versatility of this therapy and its particular relevance to issues faced by older people. The volume first reviews relevant gerontology issues that provide the broader context in which older lives are lived. Knowledge of depression and later life are then discussed in chapter 2 along with general clinical recommendations for the assessment and treatment of older adults. In chapter 3, we make a clinical and research case for why IPT is especially well-suited for older people. In chapter 4, the general structure of IPT is reviewed along with a distillation of salient research. In much of the remainder of the book we discuss how to conduct IPT, drawing on our clinical experience with older people. A chapter is devoted to common problems that arise for those who are learning IPT. The final chapter includes a summary of concluding remarks and guidance for those who want to gain further knowledge and experience in the application of IPT. The book concludes with an annotated list of resources.

Those familiar with gerontology and geropsychology may want to quickly read through chapters 1 and 2. Those unfamiliar with gerontology and geropsychology may want to read additional books on these topics listed in the resource section. We suggest that all readers interested in using IPT read

Comprehensive Guide to Interpersonal Psychotherapy (Weissman, Markowitz, & Klerman, 2000), which contains the original treatment manual and describes the application of IPT with mixed age groups and disorders and has excellent research summaries.

Perhaps the heart of this volume is the clinical cases that illustrate the use of IPT in each of the IPT four problem areas. Clinical examples provided are actual IPT cases or composites of cases. Identifying information has been changed, and names are fictitious. A case from each of the four problem areas is presented in chapter 5, which covers the initial sessions of IPT, and subsequent chapters focus on IPT's intermediate sessions for the relevant problem area. An additional case is provided in each chapter on IPT intermediate sessions. We have used dialogue and commentary to try to make the cases as clear and clinically useful as possible.

We both feel extremely fortunate to have learned how to conduct IPT and find supervision of those learning IPT to be especially rewarding. We hope that this book will generate similar enthusiasm in the reader.

ACKNOWLEDGMENTS

Colleagues and friends have supported us in the development of this book and, more broadly, in our work with interpersonal psychotherapy (IPT). It is a blessing when one's professional endeavors are a vehicle for meeting thoughtful and dedicated individuals. The field of IPT is especially rich with such persons. Geropsychology also draws to the field a cadre of individuals who derive personal satisfaction and meaning from sharing in the rich and varied lives of older adults.

I (Gregory A. Hinrichsen) thank colleagues, friends, and family for their support. Kathleen Clougherty, LCSW, and John Markowitz, MD, were both involved in my formal training as an IPT therapist over 10 years ago. Kathy has been a wonderful and wise colleague since that time. She's the best psychotherapist I have ever met. John has been supportive of my efforts to blend IPT with geropsychology and has always been available to consult on IPT professional and research issues. Myrna Weissman, PhD, who developed IPT with her late husband Gerald Klerman, MD, welcomed me into the world of IPT and encouraged my application of their therapy to older adults. John Kane, MD, chairman of the Department of Psychiatry at The Zucker Hillside Hospital, provided initial financial support for my training in IPT and has been helpful to me in many ways during my long tenure as a psychologist at Hillside Hospital. Blaine Greenwald, MD, associate chair of psychiatry and director of the Geriatric Psychiatry Division at The Zucker Hillside Hospital, has opened the door to numerous professional opportunities as he built a model continuum of care for older adults with psychiatric disorders at Hillside Hospital. Curtis Reisinger, PhD, director of psychological services at The Zucker Hillside Hospital, has been faithfully supportive of the many psychology training programs at the hospital and efforts at our institution to disseminate empirically supported treatments. Psychology externs, interns, and postdoctoral fellows at Hillside Hospital who have participated in IPT training have brought me considerable professional satisfaction as I've watched them grow as psychologists and IPT therapists to older persons. My friends in the New York Geropsychology Group have professionally and personally nourished me with their humanity and commitment to older adults. Lillian T. Buller at the Hillside Hospital library, my bibliographic friend, has retrieved numerous books and journal articles for me during the nearly 25 years I've been at the hospital.

Rob Jerome has provided unflagging support for my career in geropsychology and editorial and valuable critical commentary on almost every professional project. He made substantive and ongoing editorial comments on this book. My New York family—Rob, Rachel, and Ari—have provided loving care and understanding as I retreated to the Catskills for yet another weekend of working on this book. My mother, Kay Hinrichsen, was a model of how to live the later years with dignity and optimism. When raising six children in the 1960s, she somehow found the time to do volunteer work with older residents of the local nursing home. Her stories of those residents made them seem interesting and heroic. Through example, my mother showed me the joy that older adults can bring into one's life.

I (Kathleen F. Clougherty) owe my deepest gratitude to the late Dr. Gerald Klerman for introducing me to IPT. He was an intelligent, gifted, and kind supervisor. His knowledge of IPT and his clinical wisdom are everpresent in my work with patients and in my teaching of clinicians. After Dr. Klerman's death, John Markowitz, MD, contributed to my IPT growth and development, and we had many fine years of collaboration. My colleagues at the New York State Psychiatric Institute have been instrumental in fostering my work in IPT. Special thanks to Myrna Weissman, PhD, whose generous invitation to collaborate has led to extraordinary research, training, and supervision opportunities for me; to Laura Mufson, PhD, for expanding my IPT skills to include treatment of adolescents, and for offering me occasions to colead IPT training workshops and supervise clinicians who were interested in IPT for adolescents; and to Richard Neugebauer, PhD, with whom I have worked on numerous projects and who has generously supported my efforts in clinical research.

Two colleagues stand out in their contribution to my professional and personal growth. Greg Hinrichsen is a clinician from whom I learned as much as I taught; thank you for offering me a chance to collaborate on this book. We have spent countless hours together teaching and discussing cases and IPT concepts. It's always been a pleasure. Second, I'd like to thank Lena Verdeli, PhD, with whom I traveled to Uganda and China to introduce IPT into these cultures. Her curiosity, unwavering support, remarkable intellect, and lively sense of humor made these challenging experiences rewarding and exciting.

Hy Grossbard and Miriam Forman, PhD, helped me understand the value of the therapeutic process. I owe endless thanks to my family: Caitlin,

Mom, Dad, Connie, Bob, Brian, and Max. Thank you for your confidence in me and for listening, encouraging, pushing, and comforting me.

Finally, sincere thanks to our clients who have shared their lives with us and from whom we have learned so much.

INTERPERSONAL PSYCHOTHERAPY *for* DEPRESSED OLDER ADULTS

1

GERONTOLOGY: EXPLORING THE WORLDS OF OLDER ADULTS

We begin this book with a discussion of gerontology. Gerontologists—those who study aging—have researched the many dimensions of the lives of older adults. Gerontologists come from all the academic fields: economics, political science, social policy, psychology, sociology, biology, medicine, and the rest. What distinguishes gerontologists from others is their focus on issues related to the phenomena of aging. Gerontological sociologists study the social forces that affect older adults and how older adults have an impact on the society at-large. Gerontological psychologists are interested in how psychological phenomena vary on the basis of age. Gerontological biologists examine the biological basis of aging from insects to primates. How is gerontology relevant to mental health care professionals who want to conduct psychotherapy with older adults with depression? Gerontology provides a backdrop against which psychotherapy is provided. Gerontological research outlines the context in which individual lives are lived. Gerontology maps out the complex and sometimes contradictory forces that exist within and outside of older adults. Facts about the lives of older adults as a whole are a useful baseline against which to make sense of the individual issues an older adult brings into psychotherapy.

Those who see or plan to see older adults in clinical practice need to be familiar with gerontology, the mental health problems that exist among older adults, and psychological interventions that are useful in improving mental health problems (American Psychological Association [APA], 2004). For experienced geropsychologists, this and the next chapter are a review of salient issues in gerontology and late-life depression with an emphasis on social and interpersonal factors. Those without geropsychology background can go to the book's Resources section, where they will find recommended readings and professional resources in gerontology and geropsychology through which proficiency in geropsychology can be built.

For those providing psychotherapeutic services to older adults, two issues are key: cohort- and age-related problems. Each age cohort has unique generational experiences that, in the aggregate, shape attitudes and expectations about self, other, and world. The formative years of what newsman and author Tom Brokaw (1999) has called the "greatest generation" were lived within the context of the economic privation of the Great Depression and the challenges of a world war, the scope of which had never been witnessed in the history of humankind. Researchers have found that, in the aggregate, different generational cohorts have unique identifying personal characteristics and intellectual skills that distinguish them. Understanding the broader experiences of the generation that is now old potentially strengthens the therapeutic bond and the crafting of more sophisticated therapeutic interventions.

The current understanding of older adults does not provide a static picture. Members of the greatest generation are now quite old, and a new generation will be entering into older adulthood. As can been seen from Figure 1.1, the members of each generation or birth cohort have collectively shared experiences throughout their lives that influence their perspectives on self and world. In a similar manner, each racial or ethnic and distinct social group of older adults has historical experiences uniquely relevant to their lives. Examples include the historical relevance of Japanese internment camps during World War II for older Asian Americans and later federal apology and compensation to internees; Jim Crow laws and the civil rights movement of the 1960s for older African Americans; and, for older gay and lesbian Americans, socially and institutionally sanctioned rebuke and subsequent change of attitudes beginning with the Stonewall riots in New York. As the baby boom generation moves into its later years, the social and historical experiences that shaped its members will be concatenated with their aging lives.

The problems of older adults are often driven by health-related changes associated with aging. Older adults contend with increasing health problems, need to care for friends and loved ones with health problems, cognitive changes, economic pressures tied to reduced income because of retirement or

1939 Cohort	1929 Cohort	1919 Cohort	Year	Event
		Born	1919	Influenza pandemic ends/Treaty of Versailles
			1920	Women can vote
		5 years old	1924	
	Born		1929	Stock market crashes
	5 years old	15 years old	1934	
			1935	Social Security Act
Born			1939	
			1941	Pearl Harbor/U.S. enters WWII
5 years old	15 years old	25 years old	1944	
			1946	Baby Boom begins
			1949	
			1950	U.S. enters Korean War
15 years old	25 years old	35 years old	1954	
			1955	Polio vaccine
			1956	Women age 62-64 eligible for reduced Social Security benefits
			1957	Social Security Disability Insurance implemented
			1959	
			1961	Men age 62-64 eligible for reduced Social Security benefits
			1962	Self-Employed Individual Retirement Act (Keogh Act)
25 years old	35 years old	45 years old	1964	U.S. enters Vietnam War; Civil Rights Act; Baby Boom ends
			1965	Medicare and Medicaid established
			1969	First man on the moon
			1972	Formula for Social Security cost-of-living adjustment established
			1973	Social Security Supplemental Security Income implemented
35 years old	45 years old	55 years old	1974	IRAs established
			1975	Age Discrimination Act
			1978	401(k)s established
			1979	
			1983	Social Security eligibility age increased for full benefits
45 years old	55 years old	65 years old	1984	Widows entitled to pension benefits if spouse was vested
			1986	Mandatory retirement eliminated for most workers
			1989	Berlin Wall falls
			1990	Americans with Disabilities Act
55 years old	65 years old	75 years old	1994	
			1997	Medicare payment policies changed by Balanced Budget Act
			1999	
			2000	Social Security earnings test eliminated for full retirement age
			2001	September 11
			2003	Medicare prescription drug benefit passed
65 years old	75 years old	85 years old	2004	

Figure 1.1. The historical experience of three cohorts of older Americans: A timeline of selected events. From *Older Americans 2004: Key Indicators for Well-Being* (cover), by Federal Interagency Forum on Aging-Related Statistics (November, 2004), Washington, DC: U.S. Government Printing Office. In the public domain.

inability to work, loss of friends and family from death, and other associated difficulties. An understanding of the common problems associated with aging will help the therapist better address mental health concerns that are associated with those problems.

WHO ARE OLDER ADULTS?

Names for and definitions of persons of advanced age have shifted over the years. The year that conventionally demarcates the beginning of old age is 65. It was the criterion for judging eligibility for the first old-age pension system developed in 19th-century Bismarck, Germany. The same criterion was adopted by the United States' Social Security system in the 1930s and is often used by institutions, researchers, and the general public as a way of identifying who is old. But the U.S. Social Security eligibility criterion is changing. Individuals who are part of the baby boomer generation (those individuals born between 1946 and 1964) will not be eligible for full Social Security benefits until age 66 or 67 (Kingson & Schulz, 1997). Does this mean that 65-year-old baby boomers will no longer be considered old?

Names for persons of advanced age are many: the old, old people, senior citizens, golden agers, third agers, the elderly, elders, the aged, older Americans, older persons, older adults. This proliferation of names reflects several issues. As with any group that has been stigmatized, the naming and renaming of that group reflects efforts to counter negative stereotypes. *Senior citizens* and the *elderly* were efforts to add a little dignity to the status of being an old person. And yet even these well-intentioned titles did not quite hit the mark. The term *older adults*, increasingly used by gerontologists and geropsychologists, hedges a bit by not specifying how old is old and by indicating that persons of advanced years are adults, just as younger persons are.

But why is it necessary to underscore the fact that older persons are adults? It is likely because older persons have been characterized in ways that diminish their full adult status. Studies show that younger persons are prone to engage in patronizing speech toward older adults. Older adults themselves report sometimes they are treated by younger persons in ways that negatively stereotype them (Palmore, 2001). "You'll find out when you are old," one client playfully taunted. And the stereotypes about older adults abound. They are generally alone and lonely. They are sick, frail, and dependent on others. They are often cognitively impaired. They are depressed. They become more difficult and rigid with advancing years. They barely cope with declines associated with aging. These stereotypes come from all quarters: the general public, professionals, and even older adults themselves (APA Working Group on the Older Adult, 1998).

The term *older* permits persons of advanced (advancing?) years to determine for themselves whether they believe they belong to the world of the old. Such definitional latitude testifies to the fact that many older adults do not want to be part of that world. After all, who would want to join a club for the "depressed, demented, and dependent"? Hinrichsen directly grappled with this issue at the launch of his career in aging when he worked as a social service outreach worker to older residents of Boston's Fenway neighborhood. The outreach workers went door-to-door speaking with persons 62 years of age and older to provide information and referral to area services. Some people were shocked and offended that they had been identified as senior citizens. Research indicates that, in fact, many older adults don't see themselves as old.

Gerontological researchers have long recognized these definitional problems. To consider an aggregate of individuals that ranges from 65 years up to the maximum life span age of 120 years as one homogeneous group is certainly intellectual folly. The gerontological pie thus began to be sliced into pieces: the young old, the old, the old old, the oldest old. Yet it is recognized that even within these smaller aggregates there is considerable variability. Some 65-year-old persons with multiple medical problems have difficulty ambulating, and some 65-year-old persons take part in the Senior Olympics (Neugarten & Neugarten, 1986). In gerontology there is the maxim: The older people get, the more varied they are. It is easier to generalize about an average 18-year-old than an average 70-year-old. It is, in fact, the variability among older adults that makes the study of aging the most challenging and the most interesting of disciplines. But is gerontology a discipline or many disciplines?

AGING: PROBLEM OR PROCESS?

Is aging a problem or is it a process? Is aging normal or abnormal? The way that aging is portrayed by those who study it has real-life ramifications. Noted gerontologist Robert Butler (1975) wrote the landmark book *Why Survive? Being Old in America* in the 1970s. This powerful and thoughtful book was a polemic about society's neglect of older people in the United States. The book reflected the broader concerns of a cadre of individuals committed to increased societal support for older adults. In response to such sobering images of older adults struggling to make ends meet, a number of age-based programs were funded including the Older Americans Act that, among other things, established aging agencies in all 50 states. Senior citizen centers, senior citizen housing, and other services just for older adults were developed. Though such efforts surely improved the lot of many older Americans, some wonder whether they also reinforced the stereotype of older adults as frail and struggling. Others questioned the wisdom of making age rather than need the sole criterion for eligibility for services (Neugarten, 1982) and argued that age-based programs least benefit those most in need.

Social activism on behalf of older persons brought the establishment of the Administration on Aging and a focus on aging issues within the National Institute of Mental Health (NIMH). Much-needed resources were devoted to the study of many facets of aging, and many important contributions have been made through research sponsored by these agencies. Yet some argue that too many resources have been devoted to aging as an abnormal process and that aging is improperly equated with Alzheimer's disease (Estes & Binney, 1989). The study of resilience of older adults has been neglected.

The primary criticism is that aging has been characterized as a medical problem and not a process; that older adults are more than the sum of their infirmities; and that the social, psychological, economic, and other forces that sculpt the lives of older adults have been given short shrift.

Countervailing gerontological forces have tried to put a more positive luster on aging individuals. Only a minority of older adults have depression, dementia, or are dependant. Older adults make substantial contributions to their families and communities (Shanas, 1979). Older adults have satisfying relationships with their families and friends. Older adults demonstrate powerful capacities to cope with life's vicissitudes. These are the older adults of Tom Brokaw's greatest generation. These are the older women of the 1980s popular television program, *Golden Girls*, who date, laugh, work, and fight. Others have characterized empowered older adults in a more sinister light: The old use their voting power to make sure that their age-based entitlement programs remain even if it means that younger age groups will suffer. This age group fuels the powerful lobby, American Association for Retired Persons, to do its bidding in the halls of government. These are what some have disparagingly have referred to as greedy geezers who will bankrupt the nation. Critics of these too powerful older people demand that the young get their fair share in what has been called *generational equity* (Binstock, 1985; Binstock & Quadagno, 2001).

Apart from generational experiences, aging indeed brings with it a host of challenges, many of which are tied to health. Age brings with it, slowly or rapidly, a deterioration of the bodily organism that carries a self that is the convergence of many forces. Late life is a time of many transitions that are directly or indirectly affected by one's health or the health of other aging friends and family members. The physical environment has a greater impact than before on how life can be lived in the face of declining health and reductions in mobility associated with it (Lawton & Nahemow, 1973). Increasing health problems tap financial reserves. Health involves more than physical health; older adults face increasing risk of declines in mental abilities. Psychotherapy with a older adult with depression begins with taking stock not only of the life problems that are tied to depression but also of the resources the individual can draw on to address those problems, and the unique generational perspective through which problems and resources are viewed. This chapter discusses broad issues relevant to the lives of older adults, including demographics, health, finances, housing and the environment, and social and family relations.

DEMOGRAPHICS: IS IT OUR DESTINY?

Demographics surely seems like dry stuff to most students—the world of graphs and charts, statistics, and projections. For demographers, the size and distribution of populations are forces that shape history, a perspective that is encapsulated in the expression "demography is destiny" (Vierck & Hodges, 2003). Some countries face the challenge of population growth that just doesn't seem to stop. China and India both have populations that each exceed one billion. Many European countries face shrinking populations because death rates exceed birth rates. In many developing countries, young people constitute a sizable proportion of the population whereas in developed countries, notably those in Europe and North America, older adults are the fastest growing age group. Many factors influence the size and age distribution of populations including birth rates, death rates, and in- or out-migration. And some factors that influence population cannot be anticipated. United Nations projections for the world's population in 2050 have been revised downward by 400 million in part because of AIDS.

Because of increased attention by the media, many people in the United States have a sense that America is aging. Some assume that America is aging because older people live longer than they used to. Indeed, since 1900 persons reaching the age of 65 have gained additional years of life. In 1900, life expectancy (i.e., the number of years an individual is expected to live at a given age) at age 65 was about 77 years. In 2001 life expectancy at 65 years was about 83 years. The greatest gains, however, have been in younger years. Life expectancy at birth in 1900 was 49 years. Today life expectancy at birth is almost 80 years for women and 74 years for men. This increase reflects sharply reduced rates of childhood deaths and deaths among younger adults from infectious disease over the past 100 years. As in most developed countries, fertility rates have dropped in the United States in the past century, resulting in fewer children and a proportionally larger adult and older adult population (Federal Interagency Forum on Aging-Related Statistics, 2004). In 1900, 4% of the population was 65 years and older. Currently 12% of the population is 65 years and older (with the highest percentage of older adults in Florida, West Virginia, Pennsylvania, Iowa, and North Dakota). The fastest growing part of the older population is those 85 years of age and older (Federal Interagency Forum on Aging-Related Statistics, 2004).

One of the most formidable demographic forces in the United States is the aging of the baby boomer generation. Because of the U.S. economic depression of the 1930s and World War II, large numbers of individuals delayed having children. At the end of the war, babies began to arrive and by 1964 (the official end of the baby boom), almost 76 million individuals had been born. Some have called this boom the demographic equivalent of the "pig in the python" phenomenon. One can imagine a ball of baby boomers traveling through the length of the demographic pipeline. At the front end there were not enough pediatricians to care for all those babies or schools to educate them. As the baby boomers entered adulthood, wages were depressed by their entry into the job market and there were not enough houses for them and their newly arrived children. (Note the rise in housing prices since the late

1970s.) By the middle years, the stock market witnessed a boom and bust partly as a function of the infusion of 401(k), IRA, and other retirement monies invested by those preparing for old age. In 2011 the vanguard of baby boomers will turn 65 and by the year 2030 almost 20% of the U.S. population will be 65 years and older (Federal Interagency Forum on Aging-Related Statistics, 2004). The size of the older population will double to 70 million by 2030. As baby boomers reach the end of the python pipeline, will there be enough geriatricians or geriatric psychologists? Will there be enough nursing homes or Social Security funds to support all those older adults (Congressional Budget Office, 1993)?

The public sector ramifications of the "graying of America" have not been lost on policymakers. The U.S. Department of Veterans Affairs (VA) recognized early that it would be providing services to a large aging World War II veteran population that would begin to need specialized geriatric services in the 1980s. Indeed, many VA medical centers have the best developed geriatric medical, psychiatric, and psychological training and service delivery systems in the country. Reshaping the Social Security system before baby boomers reach retirement age has been on and off the legislative agenda for 25 years. Social Security and Medicare were the focus of the 2000 presidential campaign, and in 2005 President Bush proposed significant changes in the Social Security program. Most health care professional organizations lament the dearth of those with specialized skills to treat older adults, and there are efforts to increase the cadre of geriatric professionals and researchers (Jeste et al., 1999).

DIVERSITY IN AGING

As noted in the introduction to this chapter, there are dangers in generalizing about older adults. There is diversity within the current cohort of older adults. The vast majority (82.5%) of older adults in 2003 were non-Hispanic Whites (others include 8.4% non-Hispanic Black, 5.7% Hispanic, and 2.7% Asian). However, by 2050 non-Hispanic Whites will constitute only 61.3% of older adults (Federal Interagency Forum on Aging-Related Statistics, 2004). Life experiences and the reality of being old vary according to gender, race or ethnicity, socioeconomic status, and sexual orientation. By age 85, there are only 39 men per 100 women (Moody, 1998) because of the shorter life expectancy of men, which has led some to characterize aging as a woman's issue (Huyck, 1990). As noted earlier in this chapter, the life experiences of an older Black person can often differ sharply from those of an older White individual. Older lesbians and gay men grew into adulthood when homosexuality was criminalized and socially vilified. Some older Japanese U.S. citizens were incarcerated by their government during World War II. Within the Geriatric Psychiatry Division at Hinrichsen's institution, we serve Jewish Holocaust survivors. There is also considerable diversity within the baby boomer generation. Occupying minority group status in earlier life shapes later-life experiences in important ways.

HEALTH, PHYSICAL CHANGES, AND AGING: IF YOU'VE GOT YOUR HEALTH, HAVE YOU GOT EVERYTHING?

The expression "If you've got your health you've got everything" punctuates the view that health critically affects all aspects of life. Though this expression certainly overstates the case, it rightly underscores the importance of health issues in the lives of older adults. The one common denominator in the lives of older adults is the fact that they and their aging cohorts must increasingly contend with one and often many medical problems. Older adults actually have fewer acute illnesses than do younger adults, yet the acute illnesses they do experience can have a more adverse effect. For example, many more older adults die of respiratory infections each year than do younger adults (Vierck & Hodges, 2003). For older adults the major health challenge is chronic illness. About 80% of older adults have one or more chronic diseases. Among persons 65 years of age and older, 36% have arthritis, 50% have hypertension, and 31% have heart disease. Other chronic diseases experienced by those 70 years and older include cancer (21%), diabetes (16%), and stroke (9%; Federal Interagency Forum on Aging-Related Statistics, 2004). The prevalence of chronic conditions varies by gender, race, and ethnicity. Older women have much higher rates of arthritis and heart disease than do men. Hispanic older adults have much higher rates of arthritis than do non-Hispanic older adults. Black older adults are more likely to have diabetes, stroke, and hypertension than are non-Hispanic White or Hispanic older persons. How do older adults subjectively evaluate their own physical health? Health is generally rated well. Seventy-three percent of older persons evaluate their health as good or better; women rate their health as highly as do men. Later age and non-White race and ethnicity are associated with lower self-ratings of health (Federal Interagency Forum for Aging-Related Statistics, 2004).

A key issue is to what extent health problems impair older adults' abilities to go about their day-to-day lives. Two indicators are often used to assess these: activities of daily living (ADLs) and instrumental activities of daily living (IADLs). ADLs assess basic self-care tasks such as eating, toileting, and bathing whereas IADLs assess abilities that require basic mental competence such as paying bills, taking medications properly, and shopping. IADLs underscore the importance of mental abilities to health and daily functioning (Moody, 1998). Late-life cognitive abilities will be discussed later in this chapter. The National Long Term Care Survey found that among those 65 years of age and older, 21% had one or more ADL or IADL impairments

(Federal Interagency Forum on Aging-Related Statistics, 2000). With increasing disability, most older adults make adaptations (changing routines, using assistive devices, using help from others) to maximize functioning.

Prior to and concurrent with the advent of health problems are age-related changes in appearance, body build and shape, and senses. The appearance of gray hairs or wrinkles in the late 20s and early 30s signals the reality of the aging process. Concern and ambivalence about aging is evident throughout adulthood. Hinrichsen once gave a lecture to a group of older adults that he titled "The faces of aging." The lecture addressed the ambivalence many feel about outward signs of aging but he underscored the resilience of individuals in dealing with the challenges of aging. After the lecture an older woman approached the speaker and commented, "Thank you for coming to speak to us but I was disappointed with your lecture. When I saw that the title of your talk was 'the faces of aging,' I thought it was a lecture on makeup tips for the elderly."

FINANCES: WILL THE MONEY LAST?

In 1959 the family income of 35% of older adults was below the poverty line. Today the rate of poverty among those 65 years and older is 10%. How did this happen? Many forces have influenced the generally improved financial well-being of older adults, including the advent in the 1960s of medical insurance for older adults, Medicare, and the indexing of Social Security to inflation in the 1970s; the creation of a variety of income, food, housing, and medical support programs for low-income individuals; better retirement plans for some; and a rise in the values of assets, including housing, held by older adults. However, there is striking variation in economic well-being within the 65 years and older population (Crown, 2001). Poverty rates are higher for women than men, nonmarried than married, older than younger aged persons, and minorities than non-Hispanic Whites. Black persons 65 years of age and older have a poverty rate of 37%; for Hispanics, the rate is 44% (Federal Interagency Forum on Aging-Related Statistics, 2004). Many in this current cohort of ethnic and minority older adults enter the later years with the accumulated lifetime economic impact of low-paying jobs (some of which did not result in contributions to the Social Security system), extended periods of unemployment, and lack of access to formal retirement plans. Older people sometimes live in very different worlds because of money.

There are two major pieces of later-life economics: income and net worth. Income is money that comes in from one or more sources. Net worth is accumulated assets. The most important source of income for older adults is Social Security. Social Security accounts for two fifths of older people's total income. Asset income, pensions, and personal earnings contribute about one fifth each to the remaining total. Asset income is money that comes from investments; pensions are from former employers; and earnings are from current jobs (Moody, 1998). Over the past 40 years, fewer numbers of older adults have remained employed in the later years. One major reason is that older adults do not have to work because of improved economic circumstances. However, the primary sources of income in later life are different for less versus more economically fortunate older Americans. Older Americans in the bottom three fifths of the income distribution rely on Social Security for half or more of their income. For example, of those at the bottom one fifth, Social Security is 82% of total income. Older adults of very advanced years, women, the unmarried, and minorities have lower incomes and rely more on Social Security than do other older adults. There is concern about the economic well-being of baby boomers as they enter old age as many are not accumulating adequate retirement savings.

Net worth includes the value of real estate, stocks, bonds, and other assets. Average net worth of households headed by persons 65 years and older is $179,800. In a reflection of other economic indicators, the unmarried, minorities, and less well-educated have lower net worth. The average net worth of older Black households is only $41,000. Most of this net worth is represented by the value of their homes (Federal Interagency Forum on Aging-Related Statistics, 2004). Older adults generally remain in their homes, and reverse mortgage programs are a vehicle for tapping into home wealth for income.

The question "Will the money last?" reflects the reality that assets get depleted with advancing years, and expenses, particularly health-related expenses, increase. Money concerns of older adults are reflected in comments we hear from them. "I can't believe how much it costs to get a medical plan to supplement my Medicare." "The costs of prescription drugs will drive me to the poorhouse." "If only I had bought long-term care insurance when I was younger. I can't afford it now." "The cost of things at the supermarket grows higher and higher. Do you know what it costs to buy a tomato now?" "My house is worth so much now but I can barely afford the taxes on it." "Did you know my antidepressant medication costs $100 a month?" The specter of medical pauperization haunts some older adults. Middle- and upper-middle-class older adults purchase Medicare supplement plans that pay all or some of the costs not covered by Medicare. These plans sometimes offer limited prescription coverage. Medicare supplement plans, however, can cost several thousand dollars a year. Lowest income older adults may be eligible for Medicaid, the federal- and state-funded program for the poor. Older adults neither officially poor nor financially advantaged may find themselves spending assets to cover medical expenses. Public officials and policy analysts agree that Medicare is no longer an adequate health care plan. The new Medicare prescription drug program will offer some relief to older adults but most agree it leaves many older adults responsible for the lion's share of medication costs.

The other financial specter is the cost of long-term care. With annual nursing home costs running from $35,000 to $100,000 or more a year and the cost of a full-time home health care aide running $25,000 a year, most older adults realize that an average asset base of $179,800 will not go a long way. Spouses of older adults in nursing homes wonder what will be left for them. Some adult children worry that an anticipated inheritance will be chewed up by nursing home care. A growing industry of elder care lawyers primarily serves middle- and upper-income older adults and their families. They often work to arrange the assets of an older person so that in case of nursing home placement the older person will be eligible for Medicaid and family assets will be preserved. There are debates about the propriety of this strategy (Moody, 1998). Some ask why the general public should be held responsible for the cost of nursing homes for those who have assets that could pay for all or part. Others argue that preservation of an estate against the financial devastation of nursing home costs is legal and justifiable. Only a minority of older adults have long-term-care insurance (which often pays for nursing home and in-home care), in part because this industry is new and, in part, because the costs for insurance are very high, especially for older adults. From a governmental perspective, Medicaid was originally developed as a program for the poor but has turned into a major source of funding for nursing home care of older persons. Forty-six percent of the Medicaid budget now goes for nursing home care of older persons (Vierck & Hodges, 2003).

An issue of concern for aging baby boomers is the financial viability of the Social Security system. Social Security was established in the 1930s as a system of partial financial support for older adults, the disabled, and dependents of deceased and disabled adults. It is a pay-as-you-go system; that is, current contributors to the system pay for those receiving benefits. Although all those who pay into the system and who are eligible for benefits receive income, there is an income redistribution component. That is, lower wage workers draw more out of the system than they paid and upper-income wage earners draw out less than they paid (Kingson & Schulz, 1997; Moody, 1998).

Older adults rarely express concern about the viability of Social Security for themselves but wonder if it will be there for their children. Talk of Social Security reform has been part of public discourse since the late 1970s. In the early 1980s Social Security deductions were raised to amass a surplus to cover increased outlays when baby boomers retired. These monies were borrowed against by the federal government (and some would argue, effectively spent) in budget deficit years. In the past 10 years two bipartisan commissions have been formed to address the Social Security solvency crisis but have deadlocked on how to address anticipated deficits. Plans for partially privatizing Social Security (i.e., allowing individuals to divert a portion of Social Security contributions to private accounts) have been stymied, in part, because of the enormous costs of paying for beneficiaries who are currently in the system or who could not fully participate in the proposed privatized portion of Social Security. The issue of privatization of Social Security reemerged again in 2005. Some argue that the Social Security crisis is not a crisis at all and has been portrayed this way for political reasons (Kingson & Schulz, 1997). They propose that the crisis can be solved by reducing benefits somewhat, delaying eligibility for retirement with full benefits, and raising Social Security taxes a bit. The worst case scenario appears to be that, well into the future, the Social Security system will not be able to pay the level of benefits that is currently provided to beneficiaries.

MENTAL ABILITIES AND AGING: IS ALZHEIMER'S INEVITABLE?

Older adults sometimes joke about loss of mental ability in late life. Problems in recalling a fact or name are gently called a *senior moment* (although baby boomers are beginning to experience their share of "junior moments"). "What do you do with a memory problem?" an older woman asked one of the authors. "Forget it!" was her own joking reply. Humor about late-life mental loss reflects a common presumption that cognitive loss is part of aging. It may also be a way for older adults to cope with the fear that Alzheimer's disease or one of its clinical cousins may steal the mental processes that undergird self or the selfhood of loved ones. But there is more to the landscape of late-life mental abilities than the presence or absence of dementia. A rich literature, much of it generated by psychologists, has examined changes in mental abilities across the life span (Schaie, 1994). This body of work broadly addresses whether there are age-associated declines in mental abilities. Cognitive aging researchers have examined many aspects of mental functioning, including attention and perceptual processing, memory, and intelligence.

Psychologists who measure intelligence have long observed that average IQ scores of older adults are lower than those of younger adults. Some concluded that aging is associated with loss of mental ability. However, one cannot conclude from a cross-sectional association of aging with lower IQ scores that age causes loss of intelligence. Warner Schaie (1994) laid the methodological groundwork for studies in this area. Any apparent age-associated findings may be more a function of the cohort into which individuals were born than of age per se. Age, period, and cohort effects can, in fact, be disentangled in longitudinal studies. Older adults may have lower IQ scores because as a group they had less access to educational opportunities than did younger adults. On the basis of elegant longitudinal studies, Schaie has documented that there is relative stability in five primary mental abilities over the life course and that notable declines in those abilities do not occur until the late 60s or 70s. Two general classifications of intellectual functioning are important in understanding intellectual change over the life course: fluid and crystallized intelligence. Fluid intelligence reflects mental flexibility, the drawing of inferences, abstracting of ideas, and related concepts (Horn, 1982). For example, doing a puzzle draws on fluid intelligence. Crystallized intelligence refers to acquired knowledge through education and life experience. Vocabulary and knowledge of facts are examples of crystallized intelligence. Fluid intelligence declines significantly over adult life whereas crystallized intelligence improves. The reason why fluid intelligence declines is not known but may reflect aging of the brain. One consequence of decline in fluid intelligence is that it is harder to learn as people age and mental processes slow down. But of course the story is more complicated. Some older individuals show much greater stability in fluid intelligence than does the group as a whole. There is less decline in mental ability among the better educated, economically advantaged, and those who do mentally challenging work. Further, a number of researchers have demonstrated that declines in mental abilities can be reversed in older adults with cognitive training programs and that improvement is maintained over time (Willis & Nesselroade, 1990).

The fact that there are selective declines in mental abilities over adulthood and that notable declines only arrive well into the 60s and 70s is encouraging news. Other encouraging news is that older adults make adaptations to cognitive decline that sustain their ability to successfully function. The prevalence of dementia (i.e., progressive loss of mental ability) among those 65 years of age and older is only 5% (Raskind, Bonner, & Peskind, 2004). The less encouraging news is that with advancing years older adults are at increasing risk of clinically significant loss of mental ability. Thirty-two percent of persons 85 years and older have moderate to severe memory loss (Federal Interagency Forum on Aging-Related Statistics, 2004). The chief causes of late-life dementia are Alzheimer's disease and vascular dementia—caused by a progressive series of small strokes in the brain. Though dementia may not be inevitable, very advanced age makes it increasingly likely. Dementia is the one mental disorder for which older adults are at greater risk than younger adults (Raskind et al., 2004).

HOUSING AND THE ENVIRONMENT: FINDING SAFE HARBOR IN STORMY WATERS

There is a substantial body of research on the social and psychological effects of housing and the larger environment on older adults. Sociologist Irving Rosow (1967) found that older adults living in buildings with larger numbers of older adults were more likely to have more older friends than those living in buildings with fewer number of older adults. The explanation was that older people no longer occupy social roles (e.g., worker, parent) through which friendships are made and therefore become more dependent on the places they live to form social relationships that are more likely to develop among age peers. As people become more physically frail, the immediate environment becomes more critical to independence. The availability of an elevator in the building may make a critical difference in the kind of life one lives. Geropsychologist Powell Lawton and his colleague Lucille Nahemow posited that with decreasing competence individuals are more dependent on their environments to maintain social, physical, and emotional well-being (Lawton & Nahemow, 1973). Federal support for senior citizen housing in the 1960s and 1970s was based on the assumption that many older adults would benefit by living in housing environments that were secure, accommodated physical infirmities (e.g., elevator, bathroom grab bars, emergency call buttons), and provided social access to age peers. Monies for such housing unfortunately tended to dry up in the 1980s and managers of senior citizen housing found that over the years residents, now in their late 70s and early 80s and who moved into their buildings in their 60s, had become frail. These now very old residents needed supportive services that exceeded those that could be provided by the housing site (a phenomenon called residential aging in place; Maddox, 2001). A similar phenomenon has been observed in certain neighborhoods and apartment buildings where a group of individuals moved into them when they were young and remained into old age—sometimes referred to as naturally occurring retirement communities (NORCs). In some cities, hospitals have established on-site medical services within NORCs.

Ninety percent of persons 65 years or older reside in homes and apartments. Although some older people move elsewhere after retirement, most remain in the communities where they have spent most of their lives. Among community-residing older adults, 73% of older men live with spouses whereas 50% of older women live with spouses. These differences primarily reflect the larger number of widows than widowers in late life. Residential patterns vary by race and ethnicity (Federal Interagency Forum on Aging-Related Statistics, 2004).

As can be seen, few older people live with their adult children—an arrangement that is usually preferred by both parties. "I will never share my kitchen with anyone, not even my daughter," remarked one older woman. Older people often express a desire to remain in their homes through the end of life. However, as a person ages, the ability to remain at home depends on the kinds of health problems experienced and the availability of informal or formal care that can be provided within the home. Persons without a spouse or children are more likely to reside in nursing homes than those with one or the other. Though only 5% of persons 65 years and older reside in nursing homes, 30% of men and 50% of women will spend at least some time at the end of life in a nursing home (Hooyman & Kiyak, 1999). The authors frequently hear older adults express fear about "ending up in a nursing home," and for many family members, placement of a seriously frail older relative in a nursing home is a last resort. Proprietors of nursing homes (including for-profit and not-for-profit institutions) face the challenge of providing care to very infirm individuals, retaining competent staff, making financial ends meet, and abiding by a complex array of federal and state regulations. There is soul searching in the gerontological community about nursing homes as institutions that one nursing home expert characterized as "providing neither nursing nor a home." It is worth noting that an important setting for the provision of geropsychological services is nursing homes.

Older adults have other residential options (Maddox, 2001). Assisted living facilities provide housing for individuals who need help with personal care, meals, and recreation but who otherwise can function independently. Continuum-of-care communities are residences into which individuals typically move when they are in reasonably good health and then remain until the end of their lives. Within these communities, increased services are provided as they are needed and may include a move into a nursing home facility that is part of the care community. Assisted living and continuum-of-care residences are expensive and usually affordable only to those with financial means. Some states have adult foster care or adult family homes in which an older person with some disabilities lives with a small group of other individuals. Some healthy older adults move into private age-segregated recreational communities that offer an array of social and recreational opportunities.

SOCIAL AND FAMILY RELATIONS: WILL YOU STILL LOVE ME WHEN I'M 64?

In a classic article, "Social myth as hypothesis: The case of the family relations of old people," sociologist Ethel Shanas (1979) marshaled existing data to refute myths about the state of relations between older adults and their adult children and other family members. Common misperceptions include the notions that most older people have children who live far away; that they rarely see their children, siblings, and other relatives; and that families are not central in the care of infirm older adults. Using social science data, she refuted those myths: Most older adults have one or more children within driving distance. Most older adults see or speak with one or more children weekly. Many older people maintain active contact with siblings. The bulk of care provided to infirm older adults is provided by family members. More recent survey data finds that 88% of persons 70 years and older have regular contact with friends or neighbors, 92% have contact with non-co-residing relatives, 50% attend church, temple, or related events, and 64% are satisfied with their level of social activity (Federal Interagency Forum on Aging-Related Statistics, 2000).

In this generation of older adults, divorce is much less common than among subsequent generations. Only about 7% of those 65 years or older are divorced (although there is a trend of increasing rates of divorce among older adults). Generational social values and religious beliefs as well as economic forces account for this low rate of divorce, which stands in contrast to current rates of divorce among younger individuals that approach 50%. Does the quality of late-life marriages differ from earlier life marriages? Carstensen and colleagues (Carstensen, Gottman, & Levenson, 1995) found that older couples are more likely to engage in pleasurable activities and less likely to engage in conflict than are middle-age couples. When discussing problems, older couples are less emotionally negative and more positive than are middle-age couples. Nonetheless, for older couples, a major stressor is the onset of health problems in one member or both members. Studies of those caring for an older person with physical health problems, dementia, or depression find that caregivers experience high levels of stress and increased rates of psychiatric symptoms and syndromes (Schulz, Visintainer, & Williamson, 1990).

As baby boomers enter old age, their family profiles will differ from this generation of older Americans. Members of the baby boomer generation are more likely to have been divorced, raised children of partners of second marriages, and had biological children raised within a union between a former spouse and his or her partner. A higher percentage of baby boomers have not had children or never married compared with current and past generations of older adults. Gay and lesbian people have had long-term unions with same-sex partners and within some of these unions children have been raised (Kimmel, 2002). Some baby boomers had children as teens and others had children well into their 40s. Consistent with the ethos of this generation, more individuals have lived lives outside the bounds of societal strictures than have prior generations. For the up-and-coming group of older adults, will family relationships be closer, weaker, or just different from those of the current old? When an older baby boomer is infirm, will his or her biological child who was raised by an ex-spouse or a nonbiological child raised by the baby boomer provide care? Will existing social norms and values regarding who cares for an ailing parent endure into the next cohort of older adults? As can be seen, the social reality of the lives of older adults gets reshaped by the next group of individuals that enters into the later years.

Former mayor David Dinkins once referred to New York City as a "gorgeous mosaic." Without waxing too poetic, we believe the same can be said about each older adult's life. Different pieces of current and past demographic, health, financial, cognitive, environmental, and social parameters come together to form a unique representation. Though each late-life mosaic is different, there are commonalities among all of those crafted during the same historical period. Being aware of the individual and collective representations of older adults will help to focus the therapeutic lens on relevant life details and also broaden the lens to see the person in a larger context.

2

DEPRESSION AND OLDER ADULTS

In several intriguing articles, Gerald Klerman, Myrna Weissman (Klerman & Weissman, 1989), and their colleagues (Wickramaratne, Weissman, Leaf, & Holford, 1989) reviewed studies of depression in various age groups in several Western countries. This review suggested a number of important issues. Age groups have differential vulnerability to depression. The age cohort born after World War II appears to have earlier ages of onset of depression and higher rates of depression. In other words, age is associated with risk for depression but in a way that runs counter to the common presumption that older adults are more likely to become depressed than are younger persons. Furthermore, as current cohorts of young people reach late life, they will likely have higher rates of depression than do the current cohort of older adults. Culture and society influence risk for depression. Klerman and Weissman (1989) suggested that a number of factors may contribute to increased risk for depression among younger age groups, including increasing urbanization, greater geographic mobility with resulting loss of attachments and community, changes in family life, and changes in women's roles. Their article underscored that risk for depression is a complex biological, social, and psychological phenomenon. Their work mirrored the observation of gerontologists that social and psychological phenomena associated with membership in an age cohort are critical to understanding age-associated differences.

PREVALENCE OF DEPRESSION IN OLDER ADULTS

Until the 1980s, geriatric mental health care practitioners commonly assumed that older adults were more vulnerable to depression than were younger adults. Increased risk for depression in older adults seemed logical because they were subjected to numerous losses, including loss of health. This assumption was challenged by results from the Epidemiologic Catchment Area (ECA) study (Robins & Regier, 1991), which was the first nationwide assessment of the prevalence of psychiatric disorders in the United States. The ECA study found that older adults had, in fact, lower rates of major depression (and many other psychiatric disorders) than did younger persons. Prevalence (over 1 year) of major depression was less than 1% (0.9%) in persons 65 years of age and older compared with 2.7% in all adult age groups (ages 18–29, 2.9%; 30–44, 3.9%; 45–64, 2.3%; Weissman, Bruce, Leaf, Florio, & Holzer, 1991). Lifetime rates of major depression were also lower in those 65 years and older (1.4%) compared with all adult age groups (4.9%), despite the fact that older adults had lived more years. Lifetime rates of dysthymia were also lower in older adults (1.7%) compared with all adult age groups (3.2%).

ECA data led to a fair amount of conceptual and empirical soul-searching by geriatric researchers. Perhaps older adults have social and psychological resources that protect them from depression. Perhaps the ECA study was flawed methodologically. Perhaps depression in older adults looks different from depression in younger persons. Though subsequent studies have suggested somewhat higher rates of major depression and dysthymia in older adults than did the ECA study, researchers generally believe that, indeed, this current cohort of older persons is less vulnerable to *Diagnostic and Statistical Manual of Mental Disorders* (4th ed.; *DSM–IV*; American Psychiatric Association, 1994)[1] diagnosable major depression and dysthymia (Jeste et al., 1999). Reasons for reduced risk for diagnosable depression in older adults have been suggested. As noted in chapter 1 (this volume), historical experiences unique to each generation affect the perspectives of members of that cohort. Raised in the economic privation of the U.S. Great Depression and sobered in young adulthood by World War II, older adults had lower expectations for their lives than did subsequent generations. Collectively things turned out much better for this age cohort than expected as the United States became a dominant economic and political power in the world along with the benefits that accrued for individual citizens. As this generation entered later adulthood, medical and financial support was available that did not exist for their grandparents or even parents. Late life also turned out better than expected. Difficulties from early life enhanced these individuals' ability

---

[1]*DSM–IV* was later updated with minor revisions and published as *DSM–IV–TR*.

to cope with life difficulties, and social values and norms acquired in early adulthood have psychologically served older adults well.

As gerontologists have learned, however, generalizations about all older people tell only part of the story. Rates of major depression are much higher for older adults with health problems. Over 10% of medically hospitalized older adults, 5% to 10% of those visiting their physicians, and 12% to 20% in long-term-care facilities have major depression (Blazer, 2003). As is discussed later in this chapter, greater vulnerability to depression exists within certain subgroups of older adults than in others.

Rates of clinically significant yet nondiagnosable depressive symptoms in older adults range from 8% to 16%, and there is some evidence that depressive symptoms increase risk for subsequent diagnosable depressive syndromes (Blazer, 2003). The oldest old have higher rates of depressive symptoms than do the younger old. The *DSM–IV* includes the diagnosis of minor depressive disorder in its appendix (reflecting future consideration of minor depressive disorder as a recognized diagnostic entity). Criteria for minor depressive disorder are less stringent than they are for major depression. In part, inclusion of minor depressive disorder reflects the observation by geriatric mental health care professionals that a fair number of older adults seen in clinical practice present a symptom constellation that is not currently captured by existing *DSM–IV* criteria for major depression or dysthymia. A number of prominent geriatric mental health care researchers and clinicians believe that clinically significant depressive symptoms and minor depressive disorder should be the focus of clinical intervention. They have also expressed concern that results from ECA may lead general medical practitioners to believe that depression is a rare phenomenon in older adults.

THE PRESENTATION OF DEPRESSION IN OLDER ADULTS

Consideration of minor depressive disorder and depressive symptoms as a focus of clinical intervention mirrors long-standing questions about whether depression looks different in older than in younger adults. The second edition of the *DSM*, in fact, contained the diagnosis of involutional melancholia, thought to be a distinct depressive syndrome associated with menopause. The diagnosis was not included in *DSM–III* because of lack of evidence that it is a distinct entity. Although researchers have identified various symptom presentations that differ between old and young, a consistent picture has not emerged. Factor analyses of depressive symptoms between younger and older persons have not found major differences (Blazer, 2003). However, major depression may look somewhat different in older than in younger adults as older people may express more apathy, evidence greater irritability, make excessive physical complaints, and evidence more anxious rumination (Karel, Ogland-Hand, & Gatz, 2002). Physical complaints, however, may reflect the reality that many older adults have more health problems than do younger adults. Diagnostic assessment of older adults with medical problems can be quite challenging because physical health symptoms may overlap with psychiatric symptoms.

Some have wondered whether a first episode of depression in late life differs from earlier-onset depression. Personality problems, family history of psychiatric difficulties, and problematic marital relationships have been tied to earlier-onset depression. In recent years, researchers have found that some older adults with late-onset depression have vascular lesions in the brain, a condition called vascular depression. These individuals are at greater risk for dementia and evidence losses in executive functioning, more anhedonia, and more functional impairment (Alexopoulos et al., 1997). A late-onset depression raises the question of whether the older adult may be experiencing vascular problems.

MORTALITY AND MORBIDITY OF LATE-LIFE DEPRESSION

It is sadly ironic that though older adults have low rates of diagnosable depression compared with younger persons (Weissman et al., 1991), they have the highest suicide rates of any age group. The rate of suicide for all ages is 12.4 (per 100,000) whereas for older adults it is 21.0 (McIntosh, Santos, Hubbard, & Overholser, 1994). Some researchers believe the rate of suicide may be even higher because of reluctance on the part of family or local officials to attribute a death to suicide in an older person ("why stir things up?"). Psychological autopsy studies have found that 80% of older adults who commit suicide were depressed. The old have higher rates of suicide than do younger persons throughout the world, and rates of suicide vary widely from one country to another, reflecting the forces of culture, politics, society, and economy on risk for suicide. Reflecting these forces is the fact that despite today's relatively high suicide rate among older adults, since the 1930s suicide rates, in fact, have sharply decreased among older adults in the United States (McIntosh et al., 1994). In contrast, suicide rates have increased among teens and young adults. Some suggest that this decrease reflects improved economic circumstances for older adults since the 1930s.

A sharper focus on these data reveals that risk for suicide in older people is specific to certain subgroups. Men are at greatest risk for late-life suicide. Caucasian older adults are at much greater risk than are non-Caucasians. In fact, Caucasian men account for the majority of late-life suicides. Rates of suicide are lowest for married older people and higher for those who are single, widowed, and divorced (McIntosh et al., 1994). Other late-life risk factors include depression, past suicide attempt, substance abuse, and physical illness. Studies show that most older adults who have completed suicide had seen a physician in the prior month yet the vast majority of physicians did not ascertain that the individual was depressed or at risk for suicide (Caine, Lyness, & Conwell, 1996). When older adults try to commit suicide they often are serious about it. Among younger people, the ratio of attempts to actual completion of suicide is 30:1. In older adults it is 4:1. When older adults attempt suicide they use more lethal means than do younger persons. The chief means of committing suicide in older adults are firearms and overdose (McIntosh et al., 1994). Indirect self-destructive behaviors that may lead to suicide in older persons include obesity, smoking, alcohol, accident-proneness, and self-injurious behavior in long-term-care facilities.

A report from the Medical Outcomes Study (Wells et al., 1989) found that the functional disability associated with depression among all age groups was comparable to or greater than that in eight major medical disorders (e.g., heart disease, diabetes, arthritis). Another study concluded that major depression was the leading cause of disability in adults throughout the world (Murray & Lopez, 1996). In older adults, major depression and even depressive symptoms have been associated with physical disability (including problems in performing ADLs and IADLs; Lenze et al., 2001). Depression in older adults increases risk for the onset or exacerbation of medical problems including stroke, heart attack, hip fracture, and possibly cancer and osteoporosis. The reasons for increased vulnerability to health problems are complex and likely reflect change in health-related behaviors on the part of the older person who has depression (e.g., not taking medications, physical inactivity) and biological consequences of depression (e.g., increased cortisol levels that are associated with immune dysfunction, changes in blood platelets that are linked to heart disease). Depression is also associated with increased rates of nonsuicidal death in older adults (Blazer, 2003). Older adults with depression are also more likely to use outpatient and inpatient medical services. On the other hand, medically ill individuals are at significantly increased risk of developing major depression and depressive symptoms. Depression and medical problems often affect each other in a way that is mutually causative and may result in a downward spiral of increasing depression, leading to increasing physical health problems, and so on. Higher rates of depression among medically ill individuals have prompted efforts to educate primary medical care providers in the recognition and treatment of depression in younger as well as older adults.

VULNERABILITIES TO DEPRESSION IN OLDER ADULTS

After an examination of psychiatric, psychological, and sociological data, Michele Karel (1997) and her colleagues proposed that across the adult life span, biological, life event, and psychological vulnerabilities to depression vary by age group. Biological vulnerability to depression is quite low throughout adult life until the early 70s and then rises sharply. It is worth noting, however, that individuals with high genetic vulnerability to depression are more likely to manifest it in early life. Late-life biological vulnerability to depression includes increasing presence of medical problems, neurological disorders, and medication side effects. Stressful life events have been tied to increased risk of depression and are most common among younger adults, decrease in frequency in middle adulthood, and increase in late adulthood. Some major late-life stresses include care for an infirm older relative, medical illness in oneself, and death of family and friends. Psychological vulnerabilities are at their peak in early adulthood and decrease across the life span. Psychological vulnerabilities include certain personality characteristics, feeling of helplessness and lack of control, negative self-concept, and maladaptive coping strategies. The psychological profile of older adults is one of lower psychological vulnerabilities than younger adults and conversely more psychological strengths. Of course, psychological characteristics of each age cohort may change depending on social, historical, and related factors that collectively sculpt the psychology of each generation. Cohort-specific biological vulnerabilities may also exist. For example, higher rates of substance abuse among the baby boom generation may create biological vulnerabilities to depression when they are old.

Social and interpersonal factors—the focus of interpersonal psychotherapy (IPT)—have been tied strongly to risk for depressive symptoms and syndromes in older adults. Linda George (1994) has proposed a "stage model of social antecedents of depression" in older adults. (These are not stages in the sense of developmental theories but rather groups of variables.) Each stage represents groups of factors tied to risk for depression. Stage I includes demographic characteristics that predispose to depression. Among older adults, women and the oldest old are at greater risk for depression than are others. Substantive ethnic or racial vulnerabilities to depression in older adults do not appear to exist. Stage II is early events and achievements. Early parental divorce or separation, childhood trauma, and lower educational attainment (and some argue, very high levels of educational attainment) are associated with increased risk for depression. Stage III includes later events and achievements. Lower income, lower occupational attainment, and being unmarried are associated with depression risk in older adults. Stage IV is social integration. Individuals less involved in social or religious activities are more likely to be depressed than are those who are more involved. Stage V includes vulnerability and protective factors. For older adults physical health problems and ongoing care for an infirm older relative are documented vulnerabilities to depression whereas protective factors include the perception of adequate social support. Finally, Stage VI comprises provoking agents and coping efforts. Stressful life events and certain styles of coping with life events (coping efforts that are directed less at dealing with the life event and more at managing emotions) have been tied to increased risk of depression in older adults. Though no single factor within each stage plays a determinative role in triggering depression, they all contribute. The accumulation and interaction of factors likely add to increasing risk for depression.

THE INTERPERSONAL DYNAMICS OF LATE-LIFE DEPRESSION

An interpersonal stress that has been linked to risk of emotional distress and depression in older adults is depression in one's spouse or partner. One theory suggested that depression may be contagious for family members living with an older person who has depression (Gurland, Dean, & Cross, 1983). This theory was supported by findings of a large longitudinal study of community-residing older couples. The study documented that more depressive symptoms in one's older spouse cross-sectionally and longitudinally increased the likelihood that an older person him- or herself would be depressed (Tower & Kasl, 1995, 1996). Other studies have found further evidence of *depressive contagion* in older couples (Bookwala & Schulz, 1996; Goodman & Shippy, 2002). Spouses and adult children caring for an older adult with major depression experience high levels of subjective stress comparable to those caring for relatives with dementia (Liptzin, Grob, & Eisen, 1988). They also report contending with a number of difficulties including strain in the relationship with the older person with depression and the perception that efforts to assist the person did not seem to help (Hinrichsen, Hernandez, & Pollack, 1992). James Coyne (1976) has proposed that an interpersonal downward spiral can develop between a person with depression and a significant other, usually a spouse. At first, the spouse responds to the relative's emotional distress with attempts to relieve it. Efforts to help are rejected or do not seem to bring about the desired effect. The spouse eventually feels increasing frustration, which is directly or indirectly communicated to the relative with depression, who then feels worse. The spouse then feels guilty. Efforts to help are redoubled, bringing further frustration for the spouse, expressions of anger, and greater feelings of distress in the relative who has depression. The spouse eventually begins to disengage, which further exacerbates the relative's depression. We have observed this dynamic clinically, and research evidence supports Coyne's model of interpersonal dynamics of depression (Gotlib & Beach, 1995). Though depression can damage interpersonal relationships, those relationships can play an important role in recovery from depression. In our own research, we found that family-related issues were associated with 1-year clinical outcomes in a large group of older people who were hospitalized for major depression and whose spouse or adult children provided care (Hinrichsen & Hernandez, 1993). Findings from that research are discussed in more detail in chapter 4 (this volume). Other work has found that lack of instrumental and subjective social support in older adults treated for depression was associated with longer time to remit from depression (Bosworth, Hays, George, & Steffens, 2002; Bosworth, McQuoid, George, & Steffens, 2002).

Hinrichsen and a colleague recently reviewed research on interpersonal factors and depression in older adults (Hinrichsen & Emery, 2005). The conclusions were that (a) psychosocial factors have been cross-sectionally and longitudinally linked to risk for depressive symptoms and syndromes in older adults, (b) major depression in an older relative adversely affects other family members, and (c) a small body of research has documented the role of social and interpersonal issues on the longitudinal course of late-life depression. In chapter 3 (this volume) we summarize other evidence for the link between psychosocial factors and depression in younger age groups.

THE CLINICAL ASSESSMENT OF DEPRESSION IN OLDER ADULTS

A comprehensive mental health assessment is the first step in determining whether an older adult is depressed (Blazer, 2004). It is also a primary task of the first phase of IPT for depression. Financial pressures on institutions and independent practitioners militate against spending the amount of time many clinicians would prefer in doing an initial diagnostic and assessment intake. The tension between comprehensiveness and fiscal constraint on time becomes more acute when assessing older adults. Compared with younger persons, older adults have longer life histories and sometimes longer psychiatric histories; are often on multiple medications for several medical problems; have one or more physicians with whom contact may be necessary; and are accompanied by family members with whom the mental health care provider typically meets to gather collateral information. Clinicians find that they must do a balancing act between trying to collect a lot of information in a short time while trying to establish rapport with an older individual who may initially be reluctant to access mental health services. The mission can be accomplished but requires clarity of goals, good organization of the interview, and sensitivity to late-life issues.

One of the major tasks of the intake interview is to determine if the older adult has a *DSM–IV* diagnosable depressive disorder. The relevant disorders include major depressive disorder, adjustment disorder, dysthymia, and complicated grief. However, older adults not meeting criteria for those disorders may evidence elevated levels of depressive symptoms or meet criteria for minor depressive disorder, the diagnostic entity currently being considered for inclusion in the *DSM* psychiatric nosology. Other major domains that need to be covered in a diagnostic interview with an older or younger adult include psychiatric history, medical and medication history, cognitive functioning, current life stressors, social history (including patterns of social relationships and support, employment, education), and functional ability. We assume that the reader is familiar with the basic parameters of a mental health diagnostic and assessment intake (Blazer, 2004) and thus highlight issues that are particularly germane to assessment and treatment of older adults with depression. Older adults are assessed for depression by a range of health professionals and within a variety of settings. This discussion focuses on assessment of an older adult by a mental health care professional within an outpatient setting where IPT with older adults is usually provided. Although the basic assessment principles are common, some issues vary according to professional and setting. For example, a primary care medical doctor may be most interested in doing a quick and accurate screen for depression and then refer the client to a mental health professional. In the assessment of older adults in long-term-care facilities, issues such as privacy, confidentiality, and cognitive impairment may complicate the process. There are excellent resources that address issues in the assessment and treatment of older adults in long-term care (Molinari, 2000; Reichman & Katz, 1996).

Cohort and Communication Issues

Most older adults seek outpatient mental health evaluation or treatment at the behest of a family member. It is less common for an older adult to independently seek treatment or evaluation, and those who do are more likely to be better educated, be economically advantaged, or have a prior history of seeking mental health services. In view of that, when an assessment is being done, it is important to keep in mind that the older adult may not want to be seeing the therapist. This generation of older adults has less familiarity with mental health issues than do younger generations and may not be inclined to conceptualize life problems in psychological language. When today's older adults were young, persons with mental health problems might spend long periods in state hospitals (some forcibly committed) for treatment of psychiatric conditions that today are routinely handled on an outpatient basis. Some older people express fear that an outpatient visit is the first step on the road to institutional care. In the future, silver-haired baby boomers will be more likely to self-refer for mental health services, construct life problems within psychological frameworks, and understand from the outset the basic rationale for psychotherapy and psychiatric medications. In general, older adults' view of the doctor–patient relationship is one in which the doctor's authority is respected and the doctor is expected to directly communicate within the diagnostic or therapeutic encounter. This view may result in a failure by the older person to volunteer important information unless asked, discuss treatment options or express reservations about recommended treatments, or communicate uncertainty about what the doctor said. In contrast, baby boomers grew into adulthood when authority was questioned and a medical consumer movement developed that demanded accountability from the service provider and encouraged health care consumers (not *patients*, which connotes passivity) to take an active role in their own care.

Our child psychology and psychiatry colleagues have noted some parallels in the assessment and treatment of children or adolescents and older adults. At both ends of the age continuum, family members play an important role as informants in the assessment phase and in the facilitation of ongoing access to treatment. A major difference is that an older adult is not a minor. Despite the suggestion that in late life there is role reversal between older adults and their adult children (the parent becomes the child and the child becomes the parent), this portrayal of these late-life relationships is not accurate or respectful (E. M. Brody, 1985). Spouses and adult children often play a very important role in providing or verifying information offered by the older person. In the middle phase of IPT, especially when the problem area is interpersonal dispute, family members might be included in one or two sessions just as is done with adolescents. This information is vital when the older adult is severely debilitated by depression or is cognitively impaired. Nonetheless, discounting and negative stereotyping of older adults often play out in health care settings (Levy & Banaji, 2002). Once an older woman seen in our clinic instructed the interviewer that when her daughter was invited in to provide collateral information he should remember that she, not her daughter, was the patient. This highly accomplished but now very frail woman found it common for medical care providers to stop speaking with her or even making eye contact when her daughter entered the examining room. In such cases, request permission to invite an accompanying relative into an intake and, as recommended by our former client, maintain active engagement with the older adult during that phase of the interview.

Sensory or cognitive deficits require special attention in communication. As noted in chapter 1 (this volume), vision and hearing loss are common among older adults (Whitbourne, 1999). If there is any question about these losses, the older adult should be asked and accommodations made (e.g., "Would it be helpful if I sat closer or spoke toward your good ear?" "Could you see me better if I closed [opened] the blinds?"). Before an interview, it is wise to ask the older adult to bring needed hearing aids and glasses. Some older people are embarrassed to admit to sensory losses or are fearful to ask the care provider to make accommodations. Commercial and medical facilities are increasingly handicapped-accessible yet, some older adults who have ambulation problems tell us that some care providers have not made accommodations. As a group, older adults take longer to acquire new information so it is important to ask questions clearly and simply. For older adults with frank cognitive impairment, clarity is imperative and so is collateral information.

Medical Problems and Medications

We use a standardized hospital intake form in our geriatric outpatient clinic. In the hospital, the form is used in many different settings with clients across the age range. Geriatric clinic staff find that sometimes the form does not have enough space to list all the medical conditions and medications of incoming older clients. As noted in chapter 1 (this volume), medical problems and their associated issues are the primary challenge of late life. In a diagnostic and assessment intake with older adults, attention to medical issues is critical. Certain medical conditions (such as thyroid dysfunction) can cause depression. If the underlying medical condition is treated, the depression often improves or disappears. As noted in chapter 1 (this volume), those with medical problems are much more likely to be depressed. Certain medical problems may dictate which psychiatric medications should or should not be used. Many older adults are on many medications for health problems. The side effect of some medications is depression. Known and unknown interactions among medications may have behavioral or psychiatric effects.

The practical import of these facts for the clinician is fairly straightforward: Ask the older adult to bring in a list of medical conditions and medications to the initial interview. Use collateral sources of information if needed. With the client's written permission, contact the client's physician for a summary of his or her medication condition. Psychologists and social workers who bill services through Medicare are, in fact, required to request permission to contact the client's physician. Some clients may not have seen medical doctors in the past year or more. They should be encouraged to see a physician. Most psychiatrists will not prescribe psychiatric medications without a confident understanding of an older client's current medical problems and medications. It is useful to inquire about the temporal onset of depression in relationship to the onset of medical problems and use of medications.

Cognitive Functioning

As reviewed in chapter 1 (this volume), there is increased risk for dementia in late life, particularly among the oldest old. Those with dementia are at increased risk of depression. Therefore good cognitive screenings should be conducted. Most clinicians can get a fair sense of cognitive functioning in the course of a diagnostic interview. However, some older adults with cognitive impairment are especially skilled at covering deficits. Family members are often sensitive to subtle or not-so-subtle cognitive losses and usually are a good source of information. (Family members may also inadvertently disguise cognitive deficits by trying to answer questions posed to the older person by the clinician.) A mental status exam inquires about certain aspects of cognitive functioning. Many geriatric mental health care professionals use a brief screening tool or tools to assess cognitive status. A widely used cognitive screen is the Mini-Mental State Examination (MMSE; Folstein, Folstein, & McHugh, 1975) and its more extended version, the Modified Mini-Mental State Examination (3MS; Teng & Chui, 1987). The MMSE and 3MS are easy to administer and time efficient, and there are age, education, and ethnicity norms for the MMSE. A score on a cognitive screening tool is not determinative of dementia. It provides information about whether further assessment of cognitive status is warranted (e.g., neuropsychological testing, referral to a neurologist or geriatric psychiatrist).

Measures of Depression

It can be very helpful to use instruments that quantify depression. Items from an instrument can be used to systematically inquire about symptoms that are part of a depressive syndrome. The sum of items gives a rough sense of depression severity and then becomes a baseline against which to judge one important dimension of treatment effectiveness. In the initial sessions of IPT, ratings from instruments can be used in initial education of the client about depression. There are a myriad of depression rating scales, some of which have been used with older adults. We present the most commonly used measures for which adequate research support exists for their use with older adults.

The Hamilton Rating Scale for Depression (HRSD; Hamilton, 1960) has been widely used in research and clinical settings. As originally developed, the HRSD did not have standardized questions to be used by the interviewer to elicit responses from clients. A better structured version of the measure was developed and is recommended (Williams, 1988). However, several versions of the HRSD include different numbers of items, thus making comparison of scores among these versions more difficult.

The Geriatric Depression Scale (GDS; Yesavage et al., 1983) is a 30-item measure using a yes-or-no response format that was specifically developed for older adults. There are also shorter versions of the GDS. One version has 15 items (Sheikh & Yesavage, 1986) and another version has 5 (Hoyl et al., 1999). As many older adults have medical problems, the GDS does not include somatic items that might elevate scores for medical, not psychiatric, reasons. It can be administered by the clinician or self-administered by the client. A copy of the measure can be obtained at http://www.stanford.edu/~yesavage/GDS.html.

The Beck Depression Inventory (BDI; Beck, Rush, Shaw, & Emery, 1979) has been widely used in research studies. This 21-item measure can be administered by the interviewer or by the client. Each item has four possible responses (rated 0–3) that reflect increasing severity. Summary scores are rated as *mild* (10–19), *moderate* (20–30), or *severe depression* (31 or higher). The BDI–II is a 1996 revision of the Inventory. The BDI has been used in studies of older adults and is often used by clinical geropsychologists. The BDI and BDI–II can be obtained from the Psychological Corporation.[2]

---

[2]Psychological Corporation, 555 Academic Court, San Antonio, TX 78204; http://www.psychcorp.com

THE TREATMENT OF DEPRESSION

Depression can be treated as successfully in older adults as it is in younger persons. Sixty to seventy percent of older adults treated for an episode of major depression show significant improvement in symptoms when treated with antidepressant medication, psychotherapy, or the combination (Blazer, 2003). Improvement is usually judged by a significant reduction in depressive symptoms (often, a reduction of at least half based on standard rating scales) or because the client no longer meets diagnostic criteria for major depression. Most research findings of treatment response in older adults are from acute (short-term) studies. However, for many older and younger persons, major depression is recurrent. Fewer studies have followed older adults with depression for longer periods after acute treatment for depression. Existing studies indicate that recurrence is common in successfully treated episodes of major depression in older as well as younger adults (Baldwin, 2000). For older persons with recurrent depression, continued treatment with antidepressant medication, psychotherapy, or both appears to reduce the risk of recurrence of depression. The best evidence for continuation/maintenance treatment of late-life depression in fact comes from studies of IPT. These studies are reviewed in chapter 4 (this volume).

In 1991 the National Institutes of Health (NIH; 1991) Consensus Development Conference on Diagnosis and Treatment of Depression in Late Life was convened. NIH regularly gathers experts at consensus conferences to examine the state of knowledge related to a range of health conditions. At the 1991 depression consensus conference, NIH asked experts to examine the scientific evidence on the diagnosis and treatment of depression in older adults. In a nutshell, the consensus conference concluded that proven treatments existed for late-life depression. For many geropsychologists some statements from the conference were troubling, including the conclusion that medications and electroconvulsive therapy were the first- and second-line treatments for late-life depression with a tertiary role for psychotherapy. The consensus conference concluded that psychotherapy was moderately effective in the treatment of late-life depression. In the Psychotherapeutic Interventions for Late-Life Depression section later in this chapter, an empirical rejoinder to the consensus conference's conclusions about the efficacy of psychotherapy for late-life depression is reviewed. In 1996 a follow-up to the 1991 consensus conference was held. It was sponsored by the Geriatric Psychiatry Alliance, which was established to increase awareness of psychiatric problems affecting older adults and to advocate for their mental health needs. The 1996 follow-up conference noted the rapid growth of research evidence pertaining to late-life depression and the growing maturity of the field of geriatric psychiatry and mental health and aging. There was more emphasis on the role of psychosocial interventions for depression than in the 1991 NIH consensus conference. The most recent statement of recommendations on the treatment of life depression in older adults comes from the Depression and Bipolar Support Alliance Statement on the Unmet Needs in Diagnosis and Treatment of Mood Disorders in Late Life. The group indicated that "It is now known that antidepressant drug therapy, interpersonal psychotherapy, and the combination of medication use and psychotherapeutic intervention are as efficacious in preventing recurrent major depression in elderly patients as in younger adults" (Charney et al., 2003, p. 668). In part, these enthusiastic endorsements of combination treatment reflected favorable, recently published findings from a large longitudinal study of IPT and antidepressant medication in the treatment of late-life depression (Reynolds et al., 1999).

Somatic Treatment for Depression in Older Adults

Since the 1991 depression consensus conference, selective serotonin reuptake inhibitors (SSRIs) have become the preferred antidepressant medication in the treatment of moderate to severe depression in older adults (Blazer, 2003; Mulsant & Pollack, 2004). Prior to the development of SSRIs, older as well as younger adults often were treated with another class of antidepressant medications, the tricyclic antidepressants (TCAs). The chief problem with TCAs, particularly for older adults, is side effects. TCAs may prompt adverse cardiac changes, orthostatic hypotension (a condition in which blood pressure temporarily drops, especially when an individual stands suddenly, putting the person at risk for falling), anticholinergic phenomena (such as dry mouth, blurry vision, and constipation), and other difficulties. An overdose of TCAs can lead to death, an important concern in view of the increased risk for suicide in persons with depression. Among TCAs, nortriptyline was the TCA of choice because it had fewer side effects than did others. TCAs and SSRIs appear to be equally efficacious in older as well as younger adults. The chief advantages of SSRIs are that they have many fewer side effects than do TCAs and are not fatal in overdose. Nonetheless, some persons taking SSRIs experience side effects, including weight loss, sexual dysfunction, anticholinergic effects (especially with paroxetine), agitation, and problems sleeping. Because of the more benign side-effect profile of SSRIs relative to TCAs, medication compliance appears to be higher among older people who take them. The recent recommendation from a gathering of geriatric mental health care professionals for the pharmacological treatment of major and persistent minor depression in older adults offered the following SSRI preferences: citalopram followed by sertraline and paroxetine, with fluoxetine as an alternate. Nortriptyline was the preferred TCA and desipramine was an alternative (as cited in Blazer, 2003). For older adults who experience a first episode of major depression and who recover, 1 year of antidepressant treatment is recommended. For those with two episodes, 2 or more years of continued medication treatment is recommended; and for those with three or more episodes, 3 or more years of antidepressant medication is recommended.

Other antidepressant medications can be used with older adults when SSRIs and TCAs are not effective. One option is monoamine oxidase inhibitors (MAOIs), which have been shown to be useful in the treatment of late-life depression (Georgotas et al., 1986). The major drawback of MAOIs is that they require a restricted diet because some foods that contain tyramine (e.g., cheese, sausage) may interact with MAOIs and cause a hypertensive crisis (i.e., sudden increase in blood pressure with risk for stroke).

Another option in the treatment of severe depression is electroconvulsive therapy (ECT), which has been found to be useful in treatment studies of older adults with depression (Sackheim, 1994). ECT is usually reserved for older individuals who have not responded to antidepressant medication or for persons with very severe depression who have so neglected their health that they are in physical danger. Persons with psychotic depression usually show improvement with ECT. For most individuals, ECT treatments are followed by antidepressant medication. After an initial course of ECT, some individuals receive maintenance ECT. One drawback of ECT for older adults in particular is memory loss. Research evidence indicates that memory problems are transient and usually clear within a few weeks after ECT is completed. In our clinical work, we have found that some older adults complain that they have more enduring loss of memory after ECT than research indicates.

Psychotherapeutic Interventions for Late-Life Depression

One response to the less than enthusiastic endorsement of psychotherapy for the treatment of depression by the 1991 NIH consensus conference was from geropsychologists Forrest Scogin and Lisa McElreath (1994). They conducted a meta-analysis of 17 controlled studies of psychosocial treatments for depression for older adults. They found that the effect size of these interventions for older adults was 0.78, which compared favorably with a 0.73 effect size for psychotherapy for depression among all adult ages. They also concluded that psychosocial interventions were effective for both major depression and subclinical depressive symptoms. They suggested that in contrast to the 1991 NIH consensus conference characterization of psychotherapy as moderately effective, the data indicate it is highly effective in the treatment of late-life depression. In the following years results from other studies, notably IPT research, have generally supported their conclusion.

Six major psychotherapeutic modalities for which there is at least some research evidence have been used in the treatment of depression in older adults: cognitive–behavioral therapy (CBT), psychodynamic psychotherapy, problem-solving therapy, life review therapy, family interventions, and IPT. The research literature on IPT with younger adults is reviewed in chapter 3 (this volume) and with older adults in chapter 4 (this volume).

Cognitive therapy, behavior therapy, and the combination are perhaps the best documented treatments for late-life depression. The most widely cited studies are those conducted by Dolores Gallagher-Thompson, Larry Thompson, and their colleagues at the Palo Alto VA health facilities. In a seminal study they compared treatment effects among groups of older adults with depression who were receiving cognitive, behavior, or psychodynamic psychotherapy. After 4 months of treatment (16–20 individual sessions), 52% of all study participants remitted from major depression, and no significant differences existed among therapeutic modalities. At 1- and 2-year follow-ups, most patients who had initially remitted remained so (1 year, 83%; 2 years, 77%; Thompson, Gallagher, & Breckenridge, 1987; Gallagher-Thompson, Hanley-Peterson, & Thompson, 1990). In a group format, CBT as well as psychodynamic psychotherapy was effective in the treatment of depression in older adults (Steuer et al., 1984). In a very interesting study with patients with dementia and depression and their caregivers, Linda Teri and colleagues taught family caregivers behavioral strategies that, when applied, resulted in a significant decrease in depressive symptoms in the patients (Teri, Logsdon, Uomoto, & McCurry, 1997). Bibliotherapy, in which study participants read books on cognitive or behavioral therapy for 4 weeks, was found to have acute and long-term usefulness in decreasing depressive symptoms in older adults with mild to moderate depression (Scogin, Jamison, & Davis, 1990; Scogin, Jamison, & Gochneaur, 1989). There was clinical improvement in depressive symptoms in 66% of those receiving bibliotherapy compared with 19% for those receiving no treatment. Improvement was sustained at 6- and 24-month follow-up evaluations.

Research evidence on the efficacy of brief individual psychodynamic psychotherapy comes primarily from the Palo Alto VA studies cited earlier and a related study (Gallagher-Thompson & Steffen, 1994). As noted, these studies found that dynamic therapy was as effective as cognitive and behavioral therapies in the treatment of major depression. Also as previously cited, Steuer et al. (1984) found both psychodynamic and cognitive–behavioral group therapies equally effective in the treatment of older adults with depression. As is discussed later, brief group psychodynamic psychotherapy showed efficacy comparable to that of CBT in decreasing depressive symptoms in family caregivers to frail older adults.

Problem-solving therapy helps the client to cope with depression and the problems tied to it. In problem-solving therapy, the client identifies current problems of concern, generates solutions to the problems, evaluates the potential consequences of different solutions to problems, implements problem-solving behavior, and then evaluates the actual consequences of the problem-solving efforts. As such, it shares some characteristics with IPT. Problem-solving therapy and reminiscence therapy were implemented in group formats with older adults with major depression and were compared with a waiting list control. Participants in both the problem-solving and reminiscence therapies showed significantly greater improvement in depression than did the waiting list control. Those in the problem-solving group demonstrated significantly greater improvement than did those in the reminiscence treatment group (Arean et al., 1993). An adaptation of problem-solving therapy, problem-solving treatment in primary care, was also used a treatment modality in a very large multicenter study of improving depression outcomes in older adults with major depression or dysthymia or both who were receiving medical treatment in primary care settings (Unutzer et al., 2002). Although the study did not report the unique efficacy of problem-solving therapy, patients were given access to a depression care specialist who educated the clients about depression, encouraged treatment compliance, and, when indicated, provided problem-solving treatment in primary care. Some clients used antidepressant medication. Compared with clients who received usual care, those who received the study intervention demonstrated significantly better depression-related clinical outcomes.

Life review therapy (LRT) is an approach first suggested by well-known geriatric psychiatrist Robert Butler (1963). He posited that the process of reminiscence might facilitate a better sense of self-continuity and self-worth for older persons. LRT was not developed as a treatment for depression but rather as a means of enhancing the general well-being of older adults. A few studies have examined its usefulness for older adults with depression. Results from these studies have been somewhat mixed. One study found that LRT reduced symptoms of depression in community-residing older adults with high levels of depression (Fry, 1983) whereas another found little change in depressive symptoms in a group of homebound older people (Haight, 1988, 1992). Studies of group LRT in nursing homes have also had mixed results. In one study it decreased symptoms of depression in women 65 to 74 years old but not in those 74 years or older (Youssef, 1990). In another study, a reminiscence group in a nursing home was as effective as a current topics group in increasing emotional well-being on a happiness–depression measure (Rattenbury & Stones, 1989).

Family involvement is often an important component to providing psychological services to older adults. In our clinical practice, family therapy is typically dyadic: an older client and an adult child or an older couple. The larger field of family therapy has pretty much neglected theoretical or empirical studies of late life whereas sociological studies of family are part and parcel of the field of gerontology. However, there are clinically useful commentaries on clinical work with late-life families (King, Shields, & Wynne, 2000; Qualls, 1996). Clinical research studies of families have primarily focused on spouses and adult children caring for an older person with dementia or physical health problems. Diagnosable depressive disorders and depressive symptoms are quite high among caregivers. Major depression affects from 18% to 83% of dementia caregivers (Schulz, Visintainer, & Williamson, 1990). We reviewed dementia caregiver studies and identified nine in which depression in the family caregiver was an outcome criterion (Karel & Hinrichsen, 2000). Studies that had the most success in reducing depressive symptoms used cognitive or behavioral interventions, or both, and were targeted at reduction of depression (rather than broader goals such as reducing caregiver feelings of burden). Noteworthy among these studies are those from the Palo Alto VA research group. Behaviorally based psychoeducational classes or problem-solving classes were associated with a significant reduction in depressive symptoms in caregivers of frail older people (Lovett & Gallagher, 1988). Both individual cognitive–behavioral and psychodynamic psychotherapies demonstrated usefulness in decreasing depressive symptoms in caregivers of frail older persons (Gallagher-Thompson & Steffen, 1994). As noted earlier, Teri and her colleagues (Teri et al., 1997) taught family caregivers behavioral strategies for reducing depression in their demented older relatives. It is interesting that the intervention also was associated with reduced symptoms of depression in the caregivers themselves.

CBT has the largest body of evidence that supports its efficacy in the acute treatment of late-life depression. IPT has the largest and best designed study in the continuation/maintenance treatment of late-life depression (Reynolds et al., 1999). One cannot help but be impressed with the fact that in studies that compare CBT with brief psychodynamic psychotherapy, the latter demonstrates comparable efficacy. These findings mirror those from the broader field of psychotherapy research in which most major psychotherapeutic modalities demonstrate similar levels of efficacy. In the field of applied psychology, there has been increasing emphasis on the use of empirically supported psychotherapies—that is, those therapies that demonstrate their efficacy in well-designed, controlled studies (Chambless et al., 1996; Gatz et al., 1999). This professional emphasis has not been without its critics who feel that manual-driven, research-generated psychotherapeutic modalities limit therapeutic flexibility (Levant, 2004). A larger critique of clinical research is that study subjects are not representative of the population of individuals seen in clinical practice. In research studies, patients with psychiatric comorbidities are often excluded, and more highly motivated and educated persons tend to enter clinical research. In geriatric psychotherapy research, very old and very medically ill older adults are rarely included in studies, and there is very limited research evidence on the usefulness of psychotherapies to older nursing home residents—a major growth area in clinical geropsychology. We believe all of these critiques are substantive except for the first. We do not believe that manual-guided psychotherapy limits therapeutic flexibility. In the hands of a capable psychotherapist, IPT and other empirically supported psychotherapies provide useful guideposts that, when applied with good clinical judgment, can have favorable results.

A separate issue is how the therapist responds to the fact of aging in the client and in self (Genevay & Katz, 1990). Hinrichsen was shocked early in his career when an aging psychologist at his institution with little clinical experience with older adults casually commented that a frail older client with depression might be better off dead than live with her infirmities. That comment said much about what appeared to be the psychologist's own unease with aging. We find that discussion of aging issues with our geriatric and nongeriatric colleagues frequently elicits thoughts of deceased or living older relatives who are seen as models of successful or not-so-successful aging ("Have I got a case for you—my mother!"). We believe the best remedies for countertransferential phenomena are not only personal insight but also knowledge. Knowledge of what is normative about aging will give any thinking person pause to reflect on how his or her own understanding of aging may be a mix of misinformation and projection. Some psychologists also run the risk of making older adults into heroic, saintly figures, a perception that will inevitably be challenged by an older adult who is very challenging.

BARRIERS TO ACCESSING MENTAL HEALTH CARE SERVICES BY OLDER ADULTS

Most older adults are underserved by the mental health system. Only half of older adults who recognize they have mental health problems receive treatment from either primary care physicians or mental health care providers. Only 3% of older adults have seen a mental health care professional (Administration on Aging, 2001). Only about one third of older adults treated for depression receive adequate psychotherapy services (Wei, Sambamoorthi, Olfson, Walkup, & Crystal, 2005). Despite the fact that most older adults are seen by primary care physicians, these physicians inadequately diagnose and treat or even fail to refer psychiatrically impaired older adults to mental health care specialists (Higgins, 1994). Older adults with psychiatric problems have been treated disproportionately in psychiatric units of general adult medical hospitals rather than in outpatient settings. Though a trend exists for increased use of outpatient services to treat mental health problems in older adults, older adults represent only 6% of those receiving community-based mental health services (Administration on Aging, 2001).

A limited number of mental health care professionals have specialized geriatric training (Gatz & Finkel, 1995). Few comprehensive programs exist for the delivery of mental health services to older adults. An optimal treatment paradigm is an interdisciplinary continuum of care for older adults with mental health care services that includes outpatient, psychiatric day or partial hospital, inpatient programs, and community linkages. Particularly for older adults with chronic or persistent psychiatric problems, the ability to move throughout different levels of care in one system maximizes therapeutic outcomes. A variety of health care systems associated with the VA offer a continuum of care for older adults, yet these services are restricted to eligible, mainly male, veterans while the population of older adults is predominantly female with no military service. A few comprehensive geriatric mental health care systems exist and usually are associated with academic medical centers or schools of medicine. Long-term-care facilities are rarely able to attract an adequate number of geriatric mental health care providers and only a handful have an integrated system of interdisciplinary mental health care for their residents.

One barrier to accessing mental health services has been historically limited reimbursement for mental health care under Medicare, the federal health insurance program for persons 65 years of age and older and those with disabilities (Gatz & Finkel, 1995). Until the 1980s very severe restrictions existed on reimbursement of outpatient psychiatric services, and there was virtually no reimbursement for psychological services. Annual limits for outpatient mental health care have been eliminated but mental health services are reimbursed at only 50% for most providers. The number of inpatient days that will be reimbursed for an episode of psychiatric illness is also limited. Some very low income seniors may be eligible for Medicaid, the federal and state insurance program for the poor. States can elect to pay the older patient's portion of the Medicare fee (50%) with Medicaid funds but only a few states do. Therefore, some poor older adults have limited options for accessing mental health services as providers will not receive the full Medicare-approved fee. Many independent mental health practitioners shy away from seeing clients for whom they will receive only half of the Medicare-approved fee. Some psychologists have faced problems with their local Medicare carriers (who process claims for the Medicare program) who have arbitrarily decided that psychological services to certain patients (e.g., those with cognitive loss) will not be reimbursed or who impose limits on the number of psychotherapeutic sessions that will be reimbursed (Karlin & Duffy, 2004). The Practice Directorate and the Committee on Aging of the Public Interest Directorate of the American Psychological Association fortunately have taken active steps to educate and advocate for psychologists who have confronted these problems. The reader can refer to the Medicare Toolkit and other resources prepared by the American Psychological Assocaition's Committee on Aging, which can be obtained by writing to the Committee or online at http://www.apa.org/pi/aging/lmrp.

AVAILABILITY OF PROVIDERS OF PSYCHOLOGICAL SERVICES TO OLDER ADULTS

The anticipated growth of the older population has led to what has been called "the upcoming crisis in geriatric mental health" (Jeste et al., 1999). There are about 2,500 board-certified geriatric psychiatrists and almost 700 geropsychologists, but there is a need for an estimated 5,000 of each discipline. Others estimate the need at 7,500 geropsychologists (Gatz & Finkel, 1995). A recent survey found that only 3% of practicing psychologists provided primarily psychological services to older adults (Qualls, Segal,

Norman, Niederehe, & Gallagher-Thompson, 2002). In contrast, 69% indicated that they provided some services to older adults. However, only a small proportion of these psychologists had received doctoral or continuing education in geropsychology. The likelihood is that in the future, most psychological services to older adults will be provided by psychologists who do not have a primary focus in geropsychology (Qualls et al., 2002). These findings underscore the need for exposure to geropsychology and some experience in providing services to older adults for all or most psychologists in training during graduate school and internship. For those in practice, continuing education offerings are critical to provide optimal care to older adults. The American Psychological Association's (2004) *Guidelines for Psychological Practice With Older Adults* provides useful recommendations for those who provide psychological services to older adults.

For years it has been assumed that most psychology graduate students had little interest in providing services to older adults. Recent research has challenged this assumption. A study at our own institution found that 90% of externs and interns enrolled in doctoral professional psychology programs evidenced interest in providing services to older adults after completion of training and that 38% indicated varying degrees of interest in geropsychology career specialization (Hinrichsen, 2000).

3

INTERPERSONAL PSYCHOTHERAPY: ORIGINS, STRUCTURE, RESEARCH, AND APPLICATIONS

The foundation for interpersonal psychotherapy (IPT) was laid by Gerald Klerman and Myrna Weissman in the early 1970s. Klerman was a major figure in American psychiatry. He held prominent academic positions at the Harvard School of Medicine, Yale University School of Medicine, and Cornell University Medical College. He headed the U.S. Government's Alcohol, Drug Abuse, and Mental Health Administration. He was an accomplished psychopharmacologist and an accomplished psychotherapist. He was part of a generation of psychiatry in which psychotherapy was seen as critical to the psychiatrist's role. Among colleagues and friends he was known as an enormously creative individual and gracious mentor and teacher. Although he died in 1992, he is listed as an author of the *Comprehensive Guide to Interpersonal Psychotherapy* (Weissman, Markowitz, & Klerman, 2000) because of his central role in the development of IPT. (Clougherty was supervised by and learned IPT from Klerman.) Klerman's chief collaborator in the development of IPT was Myrna Weissman, PhD, an internationally known epidemiologist and psychiatric researcher who is currently professor of psychiatry and epidemiology at the Columbia University College of Physicians and Surgeons. Dr. Weissman was also trained as a clinical social worker. Since Dr. Klerman's death, Dr. Weissman has been an integral part of the expansion of the use of IPT for different disorders and in varied populations.

What Klerman and Weissman brought to the development of IPT was a wealth of clinical experience in the treatment of persons with depression and a sophisticated understanding of clinical research. These talents were vital to the genesis and research of IPT in an era of mental health that was quite different than it is today. In the late 1960s and early 1970s, psycho-pharmacological treatment of depression was in its infancy. The psychotherapy ethos of that era was that only long-term psychoanalytic or psychodynamic psychotherapies were useful in treating depression. Psychodynamic psycho-therapies focused on the historical antecedents of current problems. An un-derstanding of those antecedents and their intrapsychic consequences was thought to result in enduring personality change with resulting amelioration of psychiatric symptoms, including depression. Cognitive and behavioral therapies had not substantively entered into psychotherapeutic practice, and use of time-limited psychotherapies was rare. Time-limited psychotherapy was viewed as, at best, a least-favored strategy that was unlikely to have sig-nificant therapeutic results. Later, professional battles began to rage between adherents of psychopharmacology and adherents of psychotherapy. The lat-ter tended to view medication treatment of depression as mere symptom re-lief whereas the former questioned whether psychotherapy had any real use-fulness. From the vantage point of the beginning of the 21st century it may be difficult to reckon with the fact that in the early 1970s there were no large-scale, multisite investigations of the acute efficacy of either medica-tions or psychotherapy in the treatment of major depression. Knowledge about the treatment of serious depression was derived from smaller studies and clini-cal observation.

While debates continue about the role of medication and psychosocial treatments for depression, the general consensus of contemporary mental health is that medication, psychotherapy, or both are all useful. The empiri-cal and professional groundwork for this change was laid, in part, by research investigations conducted by Klerman, Weissman, and other IPT researchers.

Klerman and colleagues theoretically nested IPT within the interper-sonal school of psychiatry founded by Adolf Meyer but best known through the work of Harry Stack Sullivan (1953). Meyer, Sullivan, and others associ-ated with the school emphasized the centrality of interpersonal experiences in the genesis and amelioration of psychological problems. This approach marked a departure from psychoanalytic theory which, at that time, empha-sized the centrality of early developmental conflicts around biological drives and their enduring consequences. Seeing human problems as more than the study of the mental life of people, Sullivan and other members of the inter-personal school wove sociology and anthropology into their work and pre-saged a more transactional, person–environment understanding of mental health. Interpersonal theorists saw individuals as actively adapting to the press of life problems, bringing with them interpersonal and intrapsychic strengths and deficits developed in earlier life. In many ways, this approach and Hans Selye's (1956) work on adaptation to stress laid the foundation for the contemporary study of coping, which also views people as active players in dealing with life problems armed with greater or lesser psychological and interpersonal resources (Lazarus & Folkman, 1984). See Klerman, Weissman, Rounsaville, and Chevron (1984) and Weissman et al. (2000) for their review of relevant literatures that conceptually and empirically undergird IPT.

Empirical studies subsequent to the development of IPT have continued to document the importance of interpersonal factors in depression. A colleague and Hinrichsen recently reviewed the literature in this area (which included many excellent reviews by other authors; Hinrichsen & Emery, 2005). The following is a summary of our conclusions about interpersonal factors and depression in mixed-age groups: (a) A body of well-designed research documents that life stressors are associated with increased risk for depression (Mazure, 1998). Problems in social relationships (e.g., small social networks, few close relationships, subjective perception of inadequacy in social relationships) have been tied to depressive symptoms (Kawachi & Berkman, 2001). (b) Depression impairs social functioning (Judd & Akiskal, 2000) and depression damages social relationships (Coryell et al., 1993). However, social and interpersonal functioning may improve as depression improves (Hirschfeld et al., 2000; Judd et al., 2000). (c) Marital and family functioning are impaired among individuals with psychiatric disorders including those experiencing depression (Friedmann et al., 1997). (d) Problematic interactional patterns exist between persons with depression and significant others. As noted in chapter 2 (this volume), Coyne (1976) has offered a model of the downward interpersonal spiral that develops between a person with depression and a significant other. Research generally supports his model (Gotlib & Beach, 1995). A related body of work supports the concept of depressive contagion—that is, those living with a person with depression are more likely to become depressed themselves (Joiner, 2000). (e) Interpersonal factors affect the course of a depressive episode. The emergence of life stressors during a depressive episode and problematic marital or family relationships have been tied to poorer outcomes in depression (Keitner & Miller, 1990; Mazure, 1998). Further, research on expressed emotion has documented that critical remarks by a family member toward a psychiatrically ill relative are strongly tied to a poorer course of psychiatric illness (Butzlaff & Hooley, 1998). For example, Hooley and colleagues (Hooley, Orley, & Teasdale, 1986) found that 59% of patients treated for depression who were living with a "high expressed emotion" spouse (i.e., made a relatively high number of critical remarks) relapsed within 9 months. No patients living with "low expressed emotion" relatives (i.e., made no or few critical remarks) relapsed.

In sum, theory and evidence strongly support the proposition that interpersonal factors are integral to understanding the origins and course of depression. Life events, notably interpersonally relevant events, predispose individuals to depression. Social relationships, particularly those perceived as supportive, can play a protective role when individuals confront difficult life circumstances. Yet if an individual becomes depressed, depression damages relationships—relationships that, ironically, are tied to recovery from or risk of relapse into another episode of depression.

STRUCTURE

The imperatives of clinical research demand that a psychotherapeutic intervention be manualized—that is, the goals, structure, and techniques that are part of the psychotherapy must be clearly outlined. Guided by the manual, therapists are trained to conduct the psychotherapeutic modality by those expert in its application. Therapists' fidelity to the manual is monitored to make sure that they are indeed conducting the psychotherapy as intended. These research strictures ensure that the psychotherapeutic modality is being delivered in the same manner among therapists in the study. If the clinical research study finds that the therapeutic modality is indeed efficacious, then those who want to use it in clinical practice will know how to conduct it. These were the research issues with which Klerman and Weissman contended as they developed IPT in the early 1970s. After an initial study, IPT was adopted as one of the psychotherapeutic modalities used in the first multicenter, clinical research study of medication and psychotherapy, the National Institute of Mental Health Treatment of Depression Collaborative Research Program (Elkin et al., 1989). In this landmark clinical research study of depression, IPT had to be conducted in the same manner not only in the center where it was developed but also in clinical research centers in different parts of the country.

The IPT treatment manual was published as *Interpersonal Psychotherapy of Depression* (Klerman et al., 1984). This readable, clinically friendly book outlines how IPT is conducted and includes clinical case material. An updated volume published in 2000 as the *Comprehensive Guide to Interpersonal Psychotherapy* (Weissman et al., 2000) includes summaries of IPT research studies on depression and on the wide variety of other clinical conditions and clinical populations to which IPT has been applied.

What is described in subsequent chapters of this volume is an application of IPT as originally developed by Klerman and Weissman. Broader principles for conducting psychotherapy with older adults are woven into the discussion of IPT with older adults (see Knight, 2004) and guidance is provided to the reader on how to nest common late-life problems into the IPT framework. The clinical cases in this volume therefore illustrate a gerontologically informed application of IPT with older people. The fact that

IPT can so readily be applied to older adults attests to the versatility of this therapeutic modality. As noted earlier, those interested in conducting IPT should read the *Comprehensive Guide to Interpersonal Psychotherapy* (Weissman et al., 2000). What follows in this chapter is a broad summary of the principles outlined in *Comprehensive Guide to Interpersonal Psychotherapy* (Weissman et al., 2000).

IPT is conducted in three phases of treatment: initial sessions, intermediate sessions, and termination sessions. In the intermediate sessions, therapy is focused on one or two of four problem areas: grief (complicated bereavement), interpersonal role disputes (difficulties with a significant other), role transitions (major life changes), and interpersonal deficits (difficulties establishing or sustaining relationships). In the acute treatment of depression, IPT has been conducted typically in 16 sessions on a weekly basis. Following a course of IPT in the treatment of depression, other studies have examined the usefulness of less frequent IPT sessions (approximately monthly) to reduce the likelihood of relapse or recurrence of another episode of depression.

In IPT, clinical depression is viewed as having three primary components: symptoms, social and interpersonal relationships, and personality and character problems. IPT targets the first two components for intervention; that is, a primary goal of IPT is significant reduction in depressive symptoms and improvement in social or interpersonally relevant problems that appear associated with the onset of depression or are a result of depression. Individuals have enduring traits that are often labeled as personality such as communication styles and varying propensities to anger, guilt, and self-esteem. Problems in these domains are known to predispose a person to depression. However, IPT does not attempt to change personality or character. It is increasingly recognized that what may appear to be unproductive, enduring personality characteristics during an episode of depression may actually be part of depression and therefore may not be evident after resolution of the depressive episode. For those with enduring personality-related difficulties, in IPT the client may be taught social skills that will improve ability to relate to others.

A critical component of IPT is that depression is characterized as a medical illness or clinical disorder. This frame on the client's symptom constellation provides a structure for helping the client to understand why it is often difficult to function in social roles and relationships and, with that understanding, reduce self-blame. Within the illness framework, clients can be further educated about depression and taught to monitor symptom changes and their relationship to interpersonally relevant events and to gauge symptom improvement.

Most psychotherapies share certain similarities sometimes called general or common factors (Horvath, 1988). Differences among schools of psychotherapy usually are related to how they conceptualize the origins of the presenting problem and the techniques that are used to effect change. IPT writers have outlined what are considered distinguishing characteristics of this therapeutic modality (Weissman et al., 2000).

The focus of IPT is (a) time-limited in contrast to some psychotherapies that are open-ended, (b) on one or two problem areas in contrast to therapies in which a broad range of issues may be explored, (c) on current and not remote relationships, (d) on the interpersonal and not the intrapsychic, and (e) on changing the manner in which a person contends with problematic interpersonal issues and not on cognitions and behavior as in cognitive, behavioral, or cognitive–behavioral therapies. Though IPT recognizes that personality is part of the therapeutic picture, it is not the primary focus of treatment.

THE OUTLINE OF INTERPERSONAL PSYCHOTHERAPY

The basic structure of IPT is summarized in outline form (see Exhibit 3.1) and is reproduced with permission in this chapter. The outline identifies issues that should be addressed in each phase of treatment, the goals and strategies associated with each of the problem areas, and the specific techniques that are used throughout IPT. It is assumed that individuals conducting IPT have experience in conducting psychotherapy and will generally draw on that experience to implement IPT. In this section, we broadly comment on the IPT outline. In later chapters each phase of treatment will be reviewed in detail with reference to the relevant part of the outline, accompanied by discussion of issues germane to the application of IPT with older adults.

In the initial sessions (Weeks 1–3) the therapist reviews depressive symptoms with the client, and the relevant *DSM* syndrome (i.e., typically major depressive disorder [MDD]) is identified for the client. A symptom rating scale will yield a quantitative summary of depression severity. In a psychoeducational vein, the therapist educates the client about depression and casts it as a medical illness. Existing treatments for depression are also reviewed, including the option of taking medication. As MDD is functionally impairing, the therapist educates the client about this fact and advises that it might be helpful to reduce certain responsibilities in the short run— what Klerman and Weissman call "giving the patient the sick role." The clinician reviews an inventory of relevant present and past relationships (the *interpersonal inventory*) with the client to ascertain the presence of interpersonal difficulties and any apparent interpersonal precipitant of the current episode or interpersonal problems that were seeded as a result of the episode. With this, one or two interpersonal problems areas are identified as a focus of treatment. In Week 3, the end of the initial sessions, the client is given a recapitulation of the therapist's understanding of the client's difficulties, problem area(s), treatment goals that will be the focus of treatment, and the structure of IPT.

EXHIBIT 3.1
Outline of Interpersonal Psychotherapy for Major Depression

I. The Initial Sessions
  A. Dealing With the Depression
    1. Review depressive symptoms.
    2. Give the syndrome a name.
    3. Explain depression as a medical illness; and explain the treatment.
    4. Give the patient the "sick role."
    5. Evaluate the need for medication.
  B. Relate Depression to Interpersonal Context
    1. Review current and past interpersonal relationships as they relate to current depressive symptoms. Determine with the patient the
      a. nature of interaction with significant persons;
      b. expectations of patient and significant persons from one another, and whether these were fulfilled;
      c. satisfying and unsatisfying aspects of the relationships;
      d. changes the patient wants in the relationships.
  C. Identification of Major Problem Areas
    1. Determine the problem area related to current depression and set the treatment goals.
    2. Determine which relationship or aspect of a relationship is related to the depression and what might change in it.
  D. Explain the IPT Concepts and Contract
    1. Outline your understanding of the problem.
    2. Agree on treatment goals, determining which problem area will be the focus.
    3. Describe procedures of IPT: "here and now" focus, need for patient to discuss important concerns; review of current interpersonal relations; discussion of practical aspects of treatment—length, frequency, times, fees, policy for missed appointments.
II. Intermediate Sessions—The Problem Areas
  A. Grief
    1. Goals
      a. Facilitate the mourning process.
      b. Help the patient reestablish interest and relationships to substitute for what has been lost.
    2. Strategies
      a. Review depressive symptoms.
      b. Relate symptom onset to death of significant other.
      c. Reconstruct the patient's relationship with the deceased.
      d. Describe the sequence and consequences of events just prior to, during, and after the death.
      e. Explore associated feelings (negative as well as positive).
      f. Consider possible ways of becoming involved with others.
  B. Interpersonal Role Disputes
    1. Goals
      a. Identify dispute.
      b. Choose plan of action.
      c. Modify expectations or faulty communication to bring about a satisfactory resolution.
    2. Strategies
      a. Review depressive symptoms.
      b. Relate symptom onset to overt or covert dispute with significant other with whom patient is currently involved.

continues

EXHIBIT 3.1
(Continued)

      c. Determine stage of dispute:
         i. renegotiation (calm down participants to facilitate resolution);
         ii. impasse (increase disharmony in order to reopen negotiation);
         iii. dissolution (assist mourning).
      d. Understand how nonreciprocal role expectations relate to dispute:
         i. What are the issues in the dispute?
         ii. What are differences in expectations and values?
         iii. What are the options?
         iv. What is the likelihood of finding alternatives?
         v. What resources are available to bring about change in the relationship?
      e. Are there parallels in other relationships?
         i. What is the patient gaining?
         ii. What unspoken assumptions lie behind the patient's behavior?
      f. How is the dispute perpetuated?
  C. Role Transitions
    1. Goals
      a. Mourning and acceptance of the loss of the old role.
      b. Help the patient to regard the new role as more positive.
      c. Restore self-esteem by developing a sense of mastery regarding demands of new role.
    2. Strategies
      a. Review depressive symptoms.
      b. Relate depressive symptoms to difficulty in coping with some recent life change.
      c. Review positive and negative aspects of old and new roles.
      d. Explore feelings about what is lost.
      e. Explore feelings about the change itself.
      f. Explore opportunities in new role.
      g. Realistically evaluate what is lost.
      h. Encourage appropriate release of affect.
      i. Encourage development of social support system and of new skills called for in new role.
  D. Interpersonal Deficits
    1. Goals
      a. Reduce the patient's social isolation.
      b. Encourage formation of new relationships.
    2. Strategies
      a. Review depressive symptoms.
      b. Relate depressive symptoms to problems of social isolation or unfulfillment.
      c. Review past significant relationships including their negative and positive aspects.
      d. Explore repetitive patterns in relationships.
      e. Discuss patient's positive and negative feelings about therapist and seek parallels in other relationships.
III. Termination
  A. Explicit discussion of termination.
  B. Acknowledgement that termination is a time of grieving.
  C. Moves toward patient recognition of independent competence.
  D. Dealing with nonresponse.
  E. Continuation/maintenance treatment.
IV. Specific Techniques
  A. Exploratory.

B. Encouragement of Affect.
C. Clarification.
D. Communication Analysis.
E. Use of Therapeutic Relationship.
E. Behavior Change Techniques.
F. Adjunctive Techniques.
V. Therapist Role
A. Patient advocate, not neutral.
B. Active, not passive.
C. Therapeutic relationship is not interpreted as transference.
D. Therapeutic relationship is not a friendship.

Note. From *Comprehensive Guide to Interpersonal Psychotherapy* (pp. 22–25), by M. M. Weissman, J. C. Markowitz, and G. L. Klerman, 2000, New York: Basic Books. Copyright 2000 by Basic Books. Reprinted with permission.

During the intermediate sessions (Weeks 4–13) the therapist implements treatment within the goals and strategies associated with the relevant interpersonal problem area, using therapeutic techniques that can be applied throughout the course of IPT treatment. As noted, the four problem areas include grief, interpersonal disputes, role transitions, and interpersonal deficits. For clients with grief, the broad goals are to facilitate mourning and help the client establish interests and connections with other people to substitute for the loss. Strategies to accomplish these goals include reiteration of the therapist's observation from the initial sessions that the onset of depressive symptoms followed the loss, a reconstruction of both positive and negative aspects of the relationship to the deceased, review of events associated with the deceased's death, facilitation of positive and negative feelings, and identification of practical ways to establish new connections to activities and other people.

Treatment goals for interpersonal disputes include identifying the dispute, addressing issues associated with the dispute, and modifying interpersonal behavior or expectations about the relationship to bring about resolution of the dispute. Strategies include continuing to note the connection between the depression and the dispute as well as identifying the stage of the dispute. With an understanding of the stage of the dispute, the therapist then helps the client to clarify the scope and depth of issues tied to the dispute and options, alternatives, and resources to address issues of concern. Parallel problems in other relationships and the gains and assumptions that perpetuate them as well as ways in which the current dispute is perpetuated may be identified by the therapist.

Role transitions, as major life changes are called in IPT, are the third problem area. Goals include coming to terms with the loss of the old role, regarding the new role as more positive, and restoring the client's self-esteem as a sense of mastery related to demands of the new role increases. As with all the problem areas, the presence of depressive symptoms and their connection with the problem are emphasized by the therapist. The therapist reviews positive and negative aspects of the role that is lost and associated feelings.

Concurrent with a realistic recognition of what has been lost, the client is encouraged to take a look at opportunities that accompany the new role and to develop social supports and skills needed for the new role. Along with these steps the therapist facilitates expression of associated feelings.

Persons with interpersonal deficits experience depressive symptoms because they lack the skills needed to engage other persons in their lives or have difficulties in sustaining relationships. The goals of this problem area are a reduction of social isolation and formation of new relationships. As with the other problem areas, the presence of depressive symptoms is reviewed by the therapist and their relationship with the problem area is noted. The clinician engages the client in a substantive review of positive and negative aspects of important past relationships and repetitive patterns within them. In contrast to the three other problem areas, here the therapist actively encourages the client to discuss feelings about the therapist and draw parallels in the therapeutic relationship to other relationships. These data are then used to help the client to improve social skills which will be implemented outside of the office.

Intermittently throughout IPT the client is reminded of the number of remaining sessions. In the third and final termination phase, the end of treatment is explicitly acknowledged by the therapist and discussed. Sharing feelings about ending is encouraged. The client is educated that the end of treatment can be accompanied by feelings of loss and sadness that are normal and should not be confused with a depressive relapse. In addition, the client is encouraged to express any excitement and happiness that he or she may be feeling. The therapist then reviews treatment progress and the active role the client has played in it, future challenging issues that may be on the horizon, and how the client can successfully contend with them.

A variety of therapeutic techniques will be used at different phases of treatment. Some of them are used more frequently in addressing some problem areas than others. Most of these techniques are used in other psychotherapies and therefore are not specific to IPT. Use of the techniques is in the service of the goals and strategies outlined for the respective problem areas and some of them are used in initial sessions and the termination phase of IPT.

Exploration includes nondirective techniques in which the therapist provides support for what the client is saying, encourages further discussion of the issue, or silently listens to what the client says in a way that encourages more discussion of the topic. The therapist may also ask questions to clarify information provided by the client or follow up on a topic that may provide evidence for a therapeutic hypothesis. *Encouragement of affect* is a set of techniques used by the therapist to help the client to express affect, understand it, or manage it to aid in a better understanding of self. *Clarification* techniques are used by the therapist in the short term to help the client to be more aware of what he or she has communicated and, in the longer term, to elicit information from the client that is relevant to problems that are the focus of treatment. *Communication analysis* techniques help the client better communicate with significant others. Techniques include helping the client to make clear communications rather than indirect or ambiguous ones and pointing out that clear communications have not been made when the client feels he or she has been misperceived or has misperceived the communications of others. *Use of the therapeutic relationship* uses the client's feelings about therapy or the therapist to address issues related to the interpersonal problem area. The therapist does not use this technique as an interpretation of transference (e.g., recapitulation of relationship dynamics of earlier-life primary relationships) but as a means of pointing out parallels between patient–therapist issues and those that exist in current interpersonal problems. Use of this technique may be especially important for those individuals with interpersonal deficits who may have few individuals in their interpersonal world besides the therapist. Three *behavior change techniques* are directive techniques, decision analysis, and role-playing. Directive techniques include education, modeling, and direct help to the client to address specific practical difficulties. As a primary emphasis of IPT is on the independent functioning of the client, some caution should be exercised in use of this technique. Decision analysis helps the client to lay out parameters of a problem, generate alternatives, and examine the pros and cons of different alternatives. Role-playing is a technique in which the client, or client and therapist, practice interactions with a significant other. Role-playing provides a vehicle for clarification of the client's feeling and behaviors (including a better understanding of the perspective of the other party) and is also a vehicle for practicing an anticipated discussion with a significant other. *Adjunctive techniques* include establishing an IPT treatment contract with the client in the initial sessions (conveyance of the therapist's understanding of the client's depression), explaining the parameters of IPT as a psychotherapeutic intervention, and clarifying practical aspects of therapy including frequency, time, and duration of appointments.

IPT defines the basic parameters of the therapist's role with the client. These parameters are reflected in the general stance the therapist takes when implementing IPT: (a) The therapist is a patient advocate. (b) The therapist is active and not passive. The therapist tries to strike a balance between a high level of activity and little structure or guidance in sessions. The therapist is always cognizant of the therapeutic goals that have been established and, as needed, focuses discussion on relevant issues. (c) The therapeutic relationship is not interpreted as transference. At some point in the treatment, however, if apparent problematic interactional patterns are evident, the therapist may share these with the client to facilitate better understanding of maladaptive behavior. This technique is used sparingly in IPT. If the client has concerns about the therapist's behavior that may interfere with the progress of treatment, the client is encouraged to discuss them. (d) The therapist is not a friend. The therapist sets reasonable boundaries about sharing personal information and does not establish social and business relationships with the client.

INTERPERSONAL PSYCHOTHERAPY RESEARCH

A corpus of research studies has examined the usefulness of IPT in the treatment of a variety of disorders. In this section we briefly review the key studies of IPT in the acute treatment of depression and IPT's usefulness in preventing depressive relapse. An excellent and more detailed review of studies may be found in the *Comprehensive Guide to Interpersonal Psychotherapy* (Weissman et al., 2000). Studies of IPT in the treatment of late-life depression are examined in chapter 4 (this volume). Acute treatment studies of depression examine whether a treatment is useful in significantly reducing depressive symptoms (often 50% reduction in symptom severity is used as a criterion) or whether the client no longer meets criteria for the depressive disorder (a more stringent criterion) within a specified period. Follow-up studies have usually asked the question, "Among those who respond to acute treatment, which treatment or treatments will reduce the likelihood that the study participant will subsequently evidence notable symptoms of depression?" The most credible clinical research studies are those in which individuals are diagnosed according to specific criteria and are randomly assigned to treatments including a no- or minimal-treatment control group.

Acute Treatment Studies of Depression

Two controlled studies of IPT in the individual, acute treatment of depression have been published. The first study was the Boston–New Haven Collaborative Study of the Treatment of Acute Depression (DiMascio et al., 1979; Weissman et al., 1979). This was a 16-week study of adult outpatients with major depression. Patients were assigned to one of four treatments: weekly IPT, antidepressant (amitriptyline, a commonly prescribed antidepressant at that time), a combination of IPT and antidepressant, and a control group. Compared with the control, both participants in the IPT and the antidepressant groups improved. The combination of IPT and antidepressant was better than either treatment alone. One year later, researchers contacted study participants and found that those who had received IPT (alone or along with antidepressant) showed better social functioning than did those on antidepressant alone or those who had received placebo (Weissman, Klerman, Prusoff, Sholomskas, & Padian, 1981).

The NIMH Treatment of Depression Collaborative Research Study (Elkin et al., 1989) was the second investigation of the efficacy of IPT in the treatment of acute depression. This landmark study of the efficacy of medication and psychotherapy involved several study sites throughout the country. The study included a large number of adults with unipolar, nonpsychotic depression. Subjects were randomized to 16 weeks of one of the following study treatment conditions: CBT, IPT, antidepressant (imipramine), placebo. In initial analyses, no differences were found among any of the treatment conditions. Among the most severely depressed, those treated with IPT and antidepressant did significantly better than did those in the placebo group. However, a high rate of relapse was found among those who had initially recovered (30%–50%). The high relapse rate raised concerns that after initial treatment, continued treatments were necessary to prevent further depressive relapse. Note that in the years following publication of this study, reanalyses of the original data led to somewhat different interpretations of the findings (Klein & Ross, 1993).

Continuation and Maintenance Treatment Studies of Depression

These and other studies pointed to the problem that persons successfully treated for an initial episode of depression would subsequently have another episode of depression. The terms *relapse* and *remission* have been used in different ways by different researchers to characterize the return of depression. Researchers are inclined to use the definitions developed by the University of Pittsburgh research group: Following significant improvement of depression, continuation treatment is provided to prevent relapse. *Relapse* is a significant exacerbation of depressive symptoms in the first months following remission of symptoms after acute treatment. *Maintenance treatment* is defined as clinical services provided after sustained improvement, the goal of which is to reduce the likelihood of a recurrence (i.e., a new episode of depression). Although these definitions are somewhat arbitrary, they are useful for both researchers and clinicians as a way to conceptualize the return of depression over shorter and longer periods.

The first published study of relapse following acute treatment of depression came from research data collected as part of the Boston–New Haven Collaborative Study cited earlier (Klerman, DiMascio, Weissman, Prusoff, & Paykel, 1974). A large group of female outpatients, most of whom had major depression and who had been successfully treated with antidepressant medication (amitriptyline), was randomly assigned to (a) a weekly 1-hour session of an early version of IPT called high interpersonal contact or (b) a 15-minute weekly early version of IPT called low interpersonal contact. Within each of these two groups, subjects were then randomized to antidepressant, placebo, or no pills. Antidepressant medication was associated with the best clinical outcomes. However, improved social functioning was evident toward the end of the study in subjects treated with high-interpersonal-contact IPT. The researchers concluded that the combination of IPT and antidepressant medication appeared best in the prevention of relapse and improvement of social functioning.

A critical study on continuation/maintenance treatment of depression was conducted by Ellen Frank and associates at the University of Pittsburgh (Frank et al., 1990; Kupfer et al., 1992). Adults with recurrent depression were first treated with a combination of weekly IPT and antidepressant medication (imipramine) until they showed sustained improvement of the depression. Subjects were then randomly assigned to one of five study groups: (a) a less frequent form of IPT called *maintenance IPT* (IPT-M; IPT was tapered from weekly to monthly sessions); (b) IPT-M with a placebo pill; (c) IPT-M with antidepressant (imipramine); (d) antidepressant (imipramine); or (e) placebo pill. Those in the latter two groups also received ongoing clinical management. Subjects who received only placebo had the highest relapse rate (65%) whereas the lowest relapse rate was among subjects who received both IPT-M and antidepressant (8%). Subjects who received only antidepressant or only IPT-M stayed well longer than did those who received placebo, although medication had a more powerful effect than did IPT-M. It is interesting that in other findings from this study, therapists who delivered treatment-specific IPT—that is, in a manner most consistent with its goals—had patients who did better clinically over the course of the study (Frank, Kupfer, Wagner, McEachran, & Cornes, 1991). As is discussed in chapter 4 (this volume), the University of Pittsburgh research group has also conducted a major study of continuation/maintenance in the treatment of late-life depression.

These studies provide solid evidence of the efficacy of IPT in the treatment of acute and postacute depression. The evidence is impressive for the usefulness of both antidepressant medication and IPT in improving clinical outcomes for persons experiencing serious depression. The general conclusion of studies is that both medication and psychotherapy are useful in the treatment of depression. Despite the fact that IPT and medication reduce the likelihood of recurrence of depression, recurrence rates are still relatively high even when individuals are receiving treatment. Thus researchers are challenged to find even more effective psychopharmacologic and psychotherapeutic interventions to reduce risk of relapse and recurrence. As existing treatments cannot prevent recurrence and relapse for extended periods for many people, those prescribing psychotropic medications should use optimal therapeutic dosages based on sound research data. Psychotherapists should also use psychotherapies that have demonstrated efficacy so as to maximize therapeutic outcomes.

Use of Interpersonal Psychotherapy in Other Clinical Populations

In the years since its initial development, IPT has been applied to other clinical populations and adapted for a wide variety of problems. New applications of IPT fall broadly into two categories: for individuals with depression and for those with nondepressive disorders. Those creating and researching new applications of IPT have made revisions (some minor, some major) to the original IPT manual and have generated their own treatment manuals (a partial list of which may be found in chapter 25 of *Comprehensive Guide to Interpersonal Psychotherapy* (Weissman et al., 2000). Some researchers have used IPT without adaptation. Research evidence supports the usefulness of most of the new applications, with the notable exception of substance abuse disorders for which IPT did not demonstrate clinical efficacy. The quality of evidence varies among studies. Some applications have only pilot data collected from small samples. Many applications have one or two reasonably well conducted randomized trials. Almost all of the studies would benefit from additional studies that support the short-term usefulness of IPT and its longer term efficacy (as was done by Frank and colleagues at the University of Pittsburgh with IPT-M). That being said, we admire researchers who have undertaken the enormously demanding task of conducting clinical research trials. Recruitment and retention of patients into clinical trials are difficult. Doing clinical psychotherapy research is not for the faint of heart!

As noted earlier, IPT-M is an adaptation of IPT for longer term treatment of major depression after the initial episode has significantly improved. Conjoint treatment for patients with depression with marital disputes (IPT-CM) uses IPT techniques developed in individual therapy in the treatment of couples (Foley, Rounsaville, Weissman, Sholomskas, & Chevron, 1989). An IPT adaptation developed for the treatment of dysthymic disorder (IPT-D) addresses the problems faced by individuals with chronic depression (Markowitz, 1998; Mello, Myczowisk, & Menezes, 2001). IPT and a briefer version, interpersonal counseling (IPC), have been used in medical settings by several researchers (Browne et al., 2002; Klerman et al., 1987; Schulberg et al., 1996). A study of the use of IPT with medically ill older adults is discussed in chapter 4 (this volume). Some women may become depressed during or after pregnancy, and there may be reluctance on the part of clinicians or women themselves to use antidepressant medication because of concern about the effect of medication on the fetus or breast-feeding infants. Researchers have examined the usefulness of IPT in antepartum (Spinelli, 1997; Spinelli & Endicott, 2003) and postpartum depression (O'Hara, Stuart, Gorman, & Wenzel, 2000; Stuart & O'Hara, 1995). Because of the high prevalence of depressive disorders among adolescents that occur in the context of the many developmental transitions associated with this phase of life, individual IPT and group-focused IPT have been adapted for adolescents with depression (IPT-A; Mufson, Gallagher, Dorta, & Young, 2004; Mufson, Pollack Dorta, Moreau, & Weissman, 2004). In light of the concern about the likely increased prevalence of major depression among persons with HIV infection, Markowitz and colleagues adapted IPT for this population (IPT-HIV; Markowitz et al., 1999). A major adaptation of IPT combined with social rhythm therapy has been developed by Ellen Frank and her colleagues at the University of Pittsburgh for persons with bipolar disorder (Frank et al., 1997).

In perhaps one of the more intriguing recent applications of IPT, the therapy was shown to be efficacious in the first randomized, controlled clinical trial of psychotherapy in Africa. Researchers from the Johns Hopkins and Columbia Universities trained Ugandans who had no prior mental health experience to conduct 18 weeks of IPT treatment (2 individual sessions, 16 group sessions) of Ugandans with depression (Bolton et al., 2003; Verdeli et al., 2003). Rates of major depression for subjects in the control and IPT groups were 94% and 86% at the beginning of the study. At the end of the study, control and IPT group rates of MDD were 54.7% and 6.5%, respectively. Psychotherapy clearly had a large impact on major depression.

A recent meta-analysis of IPT studies of different depressive disorders provides a useful overview of research in this area (Mello, Mari, Bacaltchuk, Verdeli, & Neugebauer, 2005). The authors reviewed randomized clinical trials of the efficacy of IPT in the treatment of a diagnosable mood disorder (including major depression, dysthymia, and both major depression and dysthymia) that met their strict inclusion criteria. Thirteen acute and longer term studies were identified, including treatment studies by Klerman, Weissman, Frank, and colleagues reviewed earlier in this chapter. Other studies included in the meta-analysis were those conducted on older adults (which are reviewed in chapter 4, this volume), adolescents, HIV-positive men, primary care patients, and women with postpartum depression. Major findings from this meta-analysis were as follows: IPT was as effective as antidepressant medication in acute and longer term studies; IPT was more effective than placebo in acute studies; the combination of IPT and antidepressant medication was no better than antidepressant medication alone in acute and longer term studies; IPT was more effective than CBT in acute treatment; and IPT had lower dropout rates than did other treatment modalities.

IPT has also been adapted for the treatment of non–mood disorders. It is perhaps puzzling to some that a psychotherapy that was designed as a treatment of depression has been used to treat nondepressive disorders. It has been argued that it is not unusual for psychotherapies or psychiatric medications originally developed to address a specific disorder to be applied to other disorders (Weissman et al., 2000). Interpersonal factors are associated with the onset or exacerbation of a variety of psychiatric disorders, and IPT's therapeutic emphasis on addressing interpersonal issues makes sense to many clinicians. For researchers looking for a psychotherapeutic modality to test in a clinical population, IPT has been attractive to many because it is manualized and has a good research track record. Some would argue that other manualized treatments would have comparable efficacy—a position that is difficult to argue with in view of the fact that researchers have found it hard to discern large differences in efficacy among different psychotherapies. Nonetheless, clinical researchers have increasingly tried to identify which therapeutic treatments are optimal for which types of problems.

IPT has been used to treat substance use disorders (for which there was no evidence of its efficacy among a group of opiate abusers; Rounsaville, Glazer, Wilber, Weissman, & Kleber, 1983), eating disorders (Agras, Walsh, Fairburn, Wilson, & Kraemer, 2000; Fairburn et al., 1991; Wilfley et al., 1993), and anxiety disorders (Lipsitz, Markowitz, Cherry, & Fryer, 1999). Other pilot work in progress is examining the usefulness of IPT for other disorders including posttraumatic stress disorder (Bleiberg & Markowitz, 2005). It is worth noting that the means by which IPT is delivered has been adapted from its original individual, in-person form to group format (Wilfley, MacKenzie, Welch, Ayres, & Weissman, 2000; Wilfley et al., 2002) and telephone format (Donnelly et al., 2000; Miller & Weissman, 2002). Weissman (1995) has developed a patient guide to IPT that can be a companion to individual IPT treatment. In a reflection of the wider appeal of IPT beyond the American shores, IPT has been translated into a number of languages, adapted and used throughout the world.

4

INTERPERSONAL PSYCHOTHERAPY FOR LATE-LIFE DEPRESSION

Almost from the beginning of scholarly study of aging, concern has been raised about the social stresses of old age and their impact on the emotional well-being of older adults—concerns that nicely dovetail with the problem foci of interpersonal psychotherapy (IPT). Social gerontologists historically have been most concerned about the loss of social roles in later adulthood. Social roles—notably marital, parenting, and occupational roles—serve as vehicles for making and sustaining contact with others. Social norms (or expectations about appropriate social behavior) are often tied to those roles. Older people thus face a much changed interpersonal landscape without normative guidance or skills to contend with it (Rosow, 1967). These issues led some social gerontologists to characterize the later years as "roleless and normless." In the absence of social roles and norms, older adults were viewed as subject to a certain social anomie and at risk for depression. In the latter part of the 20th century, we witnessed increasing opportunities for meaningful involvements in later life, yet social vulnerabilities of later life exist for some older adults. Deteriorating health is associated with reduced mobility, more difficult access to friends and family, and the challenge of transitioning into the role of a person with medical disabilities. Health problems not only predispose individuals to depression but put pressure on marital relationships as one spouse takes on increasing caregiving responsibilities for the other spouse. A large literature has documented the adverse social and emotional impact of prolonged care for a physically or cognitively impaired relative (Schulz, O'Brien, Bookwala, & Fleissner, 1995). Older adults must contend with many late-life interpersonal losses including death of spouse, other relatives, and friends and attendant grief. Health and social stresses can also put pressure on marital relationships. These stresses may be especially problematic for marriage or partnerships in which there have been long-standing problems. Loss of established social relationships confronts older persons with the challenge of reconstituting depleting social networks—a challenge for which some older adults do not possess the necessary social or interpersonal skills. As noted in chapter 1 (this volume), research has demonstrated that older adults are more resilient in the face of these social stressors than had been assumed in the early years of gerontology. Yet a subgroup of older adults is at risk for depressive symptoms, syndromes, and other mental health problems (George, 1994; Hinrichsen & Emery, 2005).

THEORIES OF ADULT DEVELOPMENT AND AGING

The field of gerontology has offered a variety of perspectives to understand continuity and change throughout the life course. Frameworks for a theoretical and empirical understanding of childhood and adolescence have been laid from the time of Freud. Freud's theories emphasized that early developmental issues were the groundwork for concerns that would be later experienced in adulthood. Piaget (1980) offered an understanding of development in childhood. What was absent for many years was a conceptual framework for understanding the life course in its entirety. Erik Erikson (1980) proffered a theory of the life cycle that took a broad and encompassing view of life at different stages that integrated the dynamic interplay of self and others. Although his and other grand theories of development have been rightly criticized for positing that all persons go through these developmental processes, his theory laid the foundation for several generations of academic research and theory that have tried to grapple with the totality of life. Erikson suggests that there are eight stages of psychosocial development that are characterized by crises reflected in polarities. The challenge of young adulthood is intimacy versus isolation; in adulthood it is generativity versus stagnation, and in old age it is integrity versus despair. The last stage involves a reckoning of the end stage of life, with the need to make sense of one's life, and continuation of generativity to the younger generations. Other, less grand conceptual frameworks have examined how central themes or issues help to understand individuals' experience of aging. The life span self-concept has been examined from a variety of perspectives by gerontologists

(Herzog & Markus, 1999). Markus, Hooker, and colleagues have studied the importance of *possible selves*—that is, an individual's projection of self into the future (Hooker, 1999; Markus & Nurius, 1986). This mental projection includes both hoped-for and feared selves. These possible selves evolve and change over the life span. Possible selves guide and inform present behavior. McAdams (1995) posits that an individual's own "life story" is an organizing and changing framework for making sense of life and experience. Whitbourne's (1987) theory of "life span constructs" suggests that individuals hold a sense of their past, present, and future conceptions of self that are important organizing principles for their lives. Levinson (1986) offers a conceptual framework of adult development that emphasizes the key role of the many transitions persons face throughout life. In these and other theories, interpersonal relationships are central players in the conflicts and joys of life that can lead to emotional disequilibrium or equilibrium.

Levinson's conception of adult development resonates best with IPT's approach to understanding and treating depression. Work by Levinson including *The Seasons of a Man's Life* (Levinson, 1978) as well as Sheehy's (1977) book, *Passages: Predictable Crises of Adult Life*, achieved considerable popularity in the 1970s and 1980s. Their inadequate research support and the contention that the posited life stages are universal have been justifiably criticized. Nonetheless, from a clinical perspective we believe Levinson offers a framework that is compatible with the principles of IPT. Like Erikson, Levinson suggests that different eras in adulthood offer unique challenges and rewards. Individuals build life structures in different eras. Each era comes to an end and is followed by a period of transition during which the existing life structure is reshaped for the next era. Levinson posits that a theory of life structure is a way of answering fundamental questions such as "What is my life like now? What are the most important parts of my life and how are they interrelated? Where do I invest most of my time and energy? Are there some relationships—to spouse, lover, family, occupation, religion, leisure, or whatever—that I would like to make more satisfying or meaningful?" (Levinson, 1986, p. 6). The major challenge of life is "an alternating series of structure-building and structure changing (transitional) periods. . . . The task of building a structure is often stressful indeed, and we may discover that it is not as satisfactory as we had hoped" (Levinson, 1986, p. 6). Consistent with most theories of adult development and aging, interpersonal relationships and one's social role in life are central themes. IPT's role transition and grief problem areas confront an individual with fundamental challenges to existing life structures. IPT's dispute problem area represents a challenge or rechallenge to the fundamental life structure of marriage or partnership or important human relationships. IPT's interpersonal deficits problem area reflects discontent with a life structure that involves too few others in a manner that is unsatisfactory. Older adults may also contend with interpersonal skills deficits as existing life structures change and the individual does not possess the requisite skills to rebuild a satisfactory network of human relations. The experience of major depression itself is disruptive to existing life structures and the relationships tied to them (Weissman & Paykel, 1974) and may concurrently challenge one's "life story" (McAdams, 1995), "life span construct" (Whitbourne, 1987), or sense of hoped-for or feared future selves (Markus & Nurius, 1986). As noted earlier, these challenges may become especially problematic for some older adults with life-stage issues such as declining health, caregiving responsibilities and associated pressures on marital or partner relationships, widowhood, and attrition of friendships. Depression and the damage it may do to interpersonal relationships make achievement of Erikson's *integrity* all the more difficult and increase the likelihood of *despair*.

Another framework from the field of gerontology offers a useful perspective that guides our understanding of late-life depression. Lawton and Nahemow's (1973) environmental docility hypothesis posits that older adults face erosion of various competencies. Those with fewer competencies become more vulnerable to environmental press, or stresses. The result is negative affect and maladaptive behavior. They concurrently posit that a certain amount of environmental press is necessary to engage the individual; those with minimal environmental press also experience negative affect and maladaptive behavior. Therefore there is a zone of optimal environmental press (i.e., not too little, not too much) but the zone depends on the level of competence for the individual. More competent individuals can maintain positive affect and adaptive behavior in the face of higher levels of environmental press than can less competent individuals. Individuals face life circumstances with varying degrees of interpersonal competence (e.g., capacity to form and sustain relationships, contend with conflict, adapt to changing human circumstances). Within Lawton and Nahemow's framework, IPT's interpersonal problems may be viewed as environmental press. Weak environmental press may represent the interpersonal environment of an individual with no or minimal interpersonal contact as reflected in interpersonal deficits. Strong interpersonal press would include role transitions, dispute, and grief. More interpersonally competent individuals are able to remain depression-free in the face of most interpersonally relevant problems whereas those who are less competent experience major depression or depressive symptoms. As noted in chapters 2 and 3 (this volume), the insidious nature of depression, however, may erode existing competencies, making the individual increasingly prone to more or sustained depressive symptoms of major depression. Other competencies bear on depression, such as biological propensity to depression, physical competence, functioning abilities, and financial resources.

The importance of interpersonal relationships to late-life depression became apparent early in Hinrichsen's career in geropsychology. One of his first older clients had a long history of recurrent major depression. This married woman in her 70s had struggled with episodes of major depression since the birth of her first child. Subsequent to the development of antidepressant medication, acute episodes of depression were successfully treated but, after 2 or 3 years, she would have another episode. Frustrated with and saddened by their mother's ongoing episodes with depression, her adult children urged her to seek treatment in our specialized outpatient mental health program for older adults. Hoping that her condition might improve with the addition of psychotherapy, her psychiatrist referred her for psychotherapy. In the first session the woman began to complain about her husband. She said that they had had an unhappy marriage made all the more difficult by what she characterized as her husband's reckless financial ventures that created financial instability within their family. In their later years he borrowed large amounts of money from loan sharks who threatened her husband when loans were not repaid in time. Though she had seriously considered divorce throughout her marriage, she felt constrained because of her religious upbringing and also values that militated against divorce and that are characteristic of this generation of older adults. The onset of episodes followed a fairly predictable pattern. Her husband would make financial arrangements that led to an increase in conflict between her and her spouse, which was followed by an episode of depression. She said that she felt trapped, without any options to change her husband. Psychotherapy focused on her options for dealing with this difficult marital situation. In the end, she enlisted her children to put pressure on her husband to exert more financial prudence and decided to ask her husband to live in another part of the house, thus limiting contact with him. Though she concluded her husband would never change, she felt that she finally had some control of her life and in the following years did not have subsequent episodes of depression.

Other early clinical experience found that family members of older clients with depression would express their frustration over the interpersonal stresses associated with an episode of depression in the relative. They were puzzled by changes in behavior in the older relative, tended to attribute depressive episodes to a lack of effort on the relative's part, and yet were guilty about their own increasing impatience with the relative because the relative was clearly suffering.

RESEARCH FINDINGS THAT PROMPTED OUR INTEREST IN IPT FOR OLDER ADULTS

Observations from our clinical practice laid the groundwork for our research investigation of interpersonal issues in late-life depression (Hinrichsen, Hernandez, & Pollack, 1992). In a study funded by NIMH, 150 persons 60 years of age and older hospitalized for an episode of major depression and a spouse or adult child most closely involved with the older adult during the episode took part in the research. We were able to follow most of these individuals for a year to assess systematically whether they had recovered from the major depression and, if they recovered, relapsed into another episode of depression. The spouse or adult child was interviewed at the admission of the older patient so we could better understand problems associated with care of the older relative, how they coped with these problems, and their own emotional adjustment. Because study findings pointed to the importance of interpersonal issues in late-life depression, they led to an interest in the use of IPT for older adults with depression.

Family members were asked what was most difficult and most rewarding in providing care to their older relative who had depression (Hinrichsen et al., 1992). The most frequently mentioned problem was interpersonal difficulties: Attempts to motivate or reason with the older person were difficult, efforts to help seemed useless or inadequate, or efforts to help were rejected by the older person. Although family members mentioned rewards much less frequently than they mentioned difficulties, the most commonly reported reward was also tied to the relationship with the older person: The relationship had improved or been enhanced since onset of depression or there was satisfaction from seeing that one's own effort had helped the older person. The latter suggested not only that some family members had been successful in contending with the problems tied to depression in the older relative, but that the episode had strengthened ties. Among those older patients we were able to follow for 1 year, 72% had recovered from the episode of major depression (Hinrichsen, 1992). Of those who recovered, 19% had another episode of major depression. Clinical outcomes were almost identical to those of a large multicenter study of primarily younger persons with affective disorders that used the same methodology for diagnosing and longitudinally assessing psychiatric outcomes (Keller & Shapiro, 1981). A critical question in the study was, "What factors at the time of the older patient's psychiatric admission best predicted the clinical course over 1 year?" The best predictors of course of depression were select family factors. Family members who themselves evidenced more psychiatric symptoms, reported more difficulties in caring for the older patient, and had poorer physical health had patient relatives who were less likely to recover (Hinrichsen & Hernandez, 1993). Family factors also influenced the risk of suicide attempts in older patients with depression. Greater family-member psychiatric symptoms, more reported caregiving difficulties, and higher levels of strain in the patient–family member relationship were tied to suicide attempts in the year following hospital admission (Zweig & Hinrichsen, 1993). In a subset of family members, rates of a brief measure of expressed emotion (EE; the construct discussed in chap. 3 that indexes expressions of critical remarks by family members toward the patient) were documented. Rates of EE were high (40%) and were tied to 1-year clinical outcomes in the older patients in the study (Hinrichsen & Pollack, 1997). A recent study documented that rates of EE in spouses and adult children of older adults with major depression are even higher (61%) when

EE is assessed with the most comprehensive measure of EE, the Camberwell Family Interview (Hinrichsen, Adelstein, & McMeniman, 2004).

These findings mirrored those from the studies of the interpersonal dynamics of depression in younger persons and their family members that were discussed in chapters 2 and 3. They also raised a practical clinical question for providers of mental health services to older adults with depression. In view of the importance of interpersonal relationships on the course of late-life depression, what could be done to improve clinical outcomes for our older adults with depression? In the early 1990s IPT had been established as effective in the treatment of depression in younger adults but there was a sparse literature on its usefulness with older persons. Nonetheless, the structure of IPT and the four interpersonal problem areas seemed promising as a treatment for late-life depression. IPT was consistent with general recommendations for doing psychotherapy with older adults—that is, in psychotherapy with older people, treatment should be problem-focused, collaborative, and psychoeducational, particularly for this generation of older adults who have less familiarity with mental health than do younger persons (Knight, 2004).

OUR CLINICAL EXPERIENCE IN PROVIDING IPT TO OLDER ADULTS WITH DEPRESSION

Hinrichsen sought out formal training in IPT that could be applied to the treatment of older adults. As part of an IPT training program at New York Hospital–Cornell Medical Center, Clougherty supervised Hinrichsen's three initial IPT cases with older adults and subsequently provided consultation on later selected cases. Clinical experience in doing IPT with older adults in the past 10 years has proved fruitful and outcomes are consistent with clinical and research reports on younger persons with depression treated with IPT. Our clinical findings follow:

- We have found clinically that 74% of outpatient older adults with depression treated with IPT demonstrate significant clinical improvement as judged by a 50% reduction in the Hamilton Rating Scale for Depression (HRSD) scores from baseline to the end of acute IPT treatment (Hinrichsen, 1997, 1999, 2004). Diagnoses of older adults treated with IPT include major depression, adjustment disorder with depressed mood, dysthymia, and dementia with depression. During IPT treatment, some clients have been on antidepressant medication and others have not.
- In order of frequency, the primary problem-focus in treatment has been role transitions, interpersonal disputes, grief, and interpersonal deficits.

- IPT can be conducted following general guidelines for conducting psychotherapy for older adults outlined in chapter 2 (this volume) and using the original treatment manual developed by Klerman and Weissman, without any substantive adaptation.
- Most clients in IPT complete acute treatment with relatively few treatment dropouts.
- Older adults find IPT an appealing psychotherapeutic modality. Focus on current rather than historical problems and establishment of therapeutic goals for acute treatment seem to make common sense to most older people. Education about depression is usually welcome even among those who have had long histories of depression. It is sometimes surprising how few older adults have been educated about depression by prior mental health care professionals. The 16-session time frame for acute IPT treatment is appealing for most of our older clients.
- Older adults with mild cognitive impairment appear to benefit from treatment. Older adults with moderate to severe cognitive impairment appear to benefit less or not at all.
- Older adults with depression who have completed acute (i.e., 16 weeks) treatment for depression appear to benefit by less frequent psychotherapy informed by IPT principles—treatment that is consistent with the structure of maintenance IPT (Frank, 1991; Reynolds et al., 1999).
- Many psychologists-in-training appear to develop at least adequate (and in some cases, more than adequate) proficiency in the conduct of IPT with older adults with close supervision of one clinical case of 16 weeks of IPT treatment of acute depression (Hinrichsen, 2004). Clinical outcomes of trainees are comparable to those of staff. Supervision takes the form of audio- or videotaped review and discussion of each of the 16 IPT sessions preceded by an overview workshop of IPT and reading of the IPT manual (Weissman, Markowitz, & Klerman, 2000). Close supervision of three IPT cases is optimal as it helps trainees to further refine IPT techniques or remediate difficulties evident in earlier cases.

Cautions must be raised about these and other clinical observations. Clinical observations are subject to a variety of biases including clinicians' tendency to rate clinical outcomes more favorably than do objective raters. Clinical outcomes may be specific to subpopulations that are treated. Although ethnic and racial diversity exists within the geriatric outpatient clinic at our institution from which most of our cases were drawn, the majority of older IPT clients are White middle-class individuals. Cases that are assigned to IPT are those in which older adults have an interpersonally relevant problem that could be the focus of treatment and who are judged capable of engaging in weekly individual psychotherapy. Persons with chronic or only partially remitted depression or who evidence marked character pathology are less likely to be referred for IPT. In conducting IPT workshops for mental health care providers, we are sometimes reminded by workshop participants of especially challenging clients (who appear to have one or more personality disorders) whom they doubt would benefit from IPT. Though we take a hopeful stance toward the usefulness of IPT in the treatment of late-life depression, some individuals are better treated by therapeutic modalities other than IPT. Also, a minority of individuals are unresponsive to either psychopharmacologic or psychotherapeutic interventions, or the combination.

RESEARCH ON IPT WITH OLDER ADULTS

In the early 1980s an article appeared suggesting that IPT might be useful for older adults with depression (Sholomskas, Chevron, Prusoff, & Berry, 1983). The authors of the article argued that IPT seemed well-suited to older adults. On the basis of clinical experience they suggested some modifications of IPT for older adults. Session duration may need to be lengthened (for talkative older persons) or shortened for some. Dependency needs were greater than with younger clients, and more advice and support may need to be given. Some older adults have chronic problems in relationships (i.e., a poor marriage) that might be better tolerated than substantively altered. Some older adults are prone to give small gifts that, within reasonable bounds, should be accepted. The therapist should be helpful to older clients around practical issues (e.g., accessing transportation and social services).

This paper was preceded by a report of pilot data by the same research group that found that 61% of older adults with depression treated for 6 weeks with IPT and antidepressant medication demonstrated improvement in symptoms (i.e., average HRSD scores were 20.90 at beginning of treatment and 7.18 at end of treatment; Rothblum, Sholomskas, Berry, & Prusoff, 1982). This paper was notable because at that time it was an open empirical question whether older adults might benefit from psychotherapy (i.e., there were very few well-designed studies of the usefulness of psychotherapy for older adults). The writers presaged contemporary interest in the use of IPT for older adults.

There is only one randomized, controlled study of IPT in the acute treatment of major depression in older adults (Sloane, Staples, & Schneider, 1985). In the study, older adults were randomized to treatment with IPT, an antidepressant (nortriptyline), or a placebo. After 6 weeks, all three groups evidenced significant improvement in mean reduction in depressive symptoms (as judged by the HRSD and the Beck Depression Inventory [BDI]). When success was judged by a 30% improvement in the HRSD, both IPT and medication tended to be better than placebo. A fairly high dropout rate was found among older persons in the medication and placebo groups but there were no dropouts in the IPT group. In view of the high dropout rates in the medication treatment (primarily because of side effects), the researchers concluded that IPT had clear advantages in the treatment of late-life depression. One problem with this study is that data on the usefulness of IPT should have been collected at the end of 16 weeks of acute treatment, not only at week 6. Also, the number of subjects was relatively small, which made it difficult to find statistically significant differences among groups. Although at that time researchers felt that a major advantage of IPT was that subjects were less likely to drop out of treatment because of side effects of nortriptyline, the current generation of antidepressant medications (i.e., SSRIs) has fewer side effects than do tricyclic antidepressants (of which nortriptyline is a part), and thus treatment dropout may be less of an issue today. Nonetheless, the study suggested that older adults could reliably engage in this psychotherapy and benefit from it.

The most convincing data on the usefulness of IPT in the treatment of late-life depression come from The Maintenance Therapies in Late-Life Depression study conducted at the University of Pittsburgh by Charles Reynolds, Ellen Frank, and their colleagues (Reynolds et al., 1999). The goal of the study was to determine which treatment or treatments were most useful in preventing or delaying the recurrence of major depression in older adults. In this study 180 persons 60 years and older with an episode of recurrent major depression were treated initially with both IPT and nortriptyline and then eventually randomized to several study groups for the maintenance phase of the study. It is worth noting that somewhat more than half of the subjects received adjunctive medication (lithium or perphenazine) during acute treatment. Subjects were treated with at least 12 weeks of IPT and a monitored dose of nortriptyline until the HRSD score was 10 or less for 3 weeks. At that point, subjects were entered into the continuation phase of the study during which they were maintained on nortriptyline and the frequency of IPT was reduced to twice monthly. To be randomized to the maintenance phase of the study, subjects were required to evidence sustained remission of the episode of major depression for 16 weeks. Subjects were randomized to four groups: nortriptyline and IPT, nortriptyline and medication clinic (brief visits in which symptoms and side effects were reviewed), IPT and placebo, and placebo and medication clinic. Study subjects were followed for up to 3 years or until they relapsed into another episode of major depression.

Maintenance IPT for late life (IPT-LLM) was used in the phase of the study and is a somewhat modified version of IPT-M that was the psychotherapy utilized in a previous maintenance study in younger individuals with major depression (Frank, Kupfer, Wagner, McEachran, & Cornes, 1991). Modifications of IPT for older adults reflected concerns raised by Sholomskas et al. (1983). In our judgment, the modifications generally reflect the kind of flexibility that is recommended in doing psychotherapy with older adults. This study showed that IPT could be conducted in a fashion parallel to its use with younger adults (Miller & Silberman, 1996). The purpose of maintenance IPT is to delay or prevent recurrence of a depressive episode. The focus of maintenance IPT is different than that of acute IPT as it is delivered monthly instead of weekly, yet it is informed by the same goals and strategies as those used in acute IPT. Whereas in acute IPT one or two problem areas are the focus of treatment, in IPT-M problem areas may shift on the basis of issues that arise for the client (Frank, 1991). The *Manual for the Adaptation of Interpersonal Psychotherapy to Maintenance Treatment of Recurrent Depression in Late Life* (IPT–LLM) is unpublished but the reader may contact the author of the manual, Dr. Ellen Frank.[1]

It is important to emphasize that older subjects in this study had significant histories of recurrent major depression with a mean HRSD score of 22, which indicates *significant depression*. In fact, they had a median of almost five lifetime episodes and 16% had a history of suicide attempts. Study findings were impressive:

- With combined IPT and nortriptyline treatment, 78% achieved remission of the episode of major depression, which attests to the usefulness of these treatments for older adults. Recurrence rates during the maintenance phase of the study were the following: nortriptyline plus IPT, 20%; nortriptyline plus medication clinic, 43%; IPT plus placebo, 64%; and medication clinic plus placebo, 90%.
- All active treatments were significantly better than placebo was. The combination of IPT and nortriptyline demonstrated a strong statistical trend for better outcomes than did nortriptyline alone. It is striking that the vast majority of older adults on placebo and medication clinic had a recurrence of major depression, which attests to the importance of ongoing treatment for older adults with recurrent depression.
- Older study subjects (70 years and older) had higher rates of recurrence than did younger old subjects. Among the older group, only those who received both IPT and nortriptyline maintained remission from the initial episode of depression.
- Subjects with lower HRSD scores (less than 20) were generally able to sustain remission on maintenance IPT (plus placebo). In contrast, those with scores higher than 20 required both IPT and nortriptyline to maintain remission.
- Those who remitted from the acute episode rapidly (within 4–5 weeks) were able to maintain remission on either IPT alone

---

[1]Ellen Frank, PhD, Western Psychiatric Institute and Clinic, 3811 O'Hara Street, Pittsburgh, PA 15213.

or nortriptyline alone in contrast to those who took longer to remit, who required both IPT and nortriptyline to maintain remission.

- Those who received both IPT and nortriptyline during the maintenance phase demonstrated better social adjustment than did those receiving only IPT or nortriptyline (Lenze et al., 2002).
- The most common IPT problem foci among study subjects included role transitions (43%), interpersonal disputes (37%), grief (19%), and interpersonal deficits (2%). More than half of subjects (57%) had a second IPT problem foci. Treatment outcomes were not related to the problem focus area (Wolfson et al., 1997).
- In comparison to findings from a parallel study of maintenance treatment of depression in younger adults, older adults achieved rates of remission from acute symptoms of major depression that were comparable to those of younger adults. However, they took somewhat longer to achieve remission and were somewhat more prone to relapse during the continuation phase of treatment (Reynolds et al., 1996).

In interpreting findings, the researchers noted that the psychotherapy effect in their study was particularly impressive in view of the fact that the maximum dose of nortriptyline was given during the maintenance phase while the minimum dose of IPT was provided (i.e., monthly). An empirical question is whether more frequent sessions of IPT during maintenance treatment of depression would result in even better psychotherapy outcomes. Study researchers concluded in their paper, published in the *Journal of the American Medical Association*, "Hence, we recommend that all older patients with recurrent depression be referred for psychotherapy, even if the pharmacotherapy is managed by the primary care physician" (Reynolds et al., 1999, p. 45). This conclusion from highly respected researchers, published in one of the premier medical journals in the country, provided unambiguous support for the role of psychotherapy in the treatment of late-life depression.

Interpersonal Counseling (IPC) is a briefer version of IPT that was developed for use in medical settings (Klerman et al., 1987). Mossey and colleagues used an adapted version of IPC in a study of subdysthymic depression in medically ill older adults (Mossey, Knott, Higgins, & Talerico, 1996). *Subdysthymic depression* refers to mild–moderate depressive symptoms that do not meet criteria for major depression or dysthymia. As noted in chapter 2 (this volume), increasing concern has been voiced about the fairly high presence of depressive symptoms in older adults—symptoms that represent increased risk for the onset of a diagnosable depressive disorder (Blazer, 2003). Medically ill older adults have elevated rates of depressive symptoms as well as much higher rates of depressive disorders compared with non–medically ill older adults. In their study, older adults who had been hospitalized for medical problems were randomized to IPC or *usual care* (in which participants rarely received formal mental health services). IPC was provided for up to 10 sessions (for 60 minutes) in a flexible manner based on medical status, with most participants receiving four or more sessions. Depression symptoms were measured at study entry with the Geriatric Depression Scale (GDS; reviewed in chap. 2, this volume), 3 months, and 6 months. Symptoms of depression were also measured in a comparison group of medically ill older adults judged to have few symptoms of depression at the beginning of the study. At 3 and 6 months, little change in depressive symptoms was evident in the comparison group whereas the usual care and IPC groups experienced reductions of symptoms. Though the IPC group had greater reduction in depressive symptoms at 3 months than did the usual care group, the differences were not significant. (It is worth noting that most older adults in the IPC group had not yet completed IPC at the time of this assessment.) However, at 6 months, the IPC group demonstrated significantly lower rates of depressive symptoms than did the usual care group. At 6 months, 61% of the IPC study patients had GDS scores less than 11 compared with only 35% of the usual care group.

SUMMARY AND CONCLUSION

IPT appears especially well-suited to older adults. Its collaborative, educational, and supportive ethos is consistent with general guidelines for conducting psychotherapy with older adults. Its four problem foci, particularly role transitions, interpersonal disputes, and grief, broadly reflect the kinds of problems many older adults confront. Our clinical experience in providing IPT in an outpatient geriatric mental health clinic suggests that clinical outcomes are comparable to those found in research studies, that there are relatively few treatment dropouts, and that many clinical psychology trainees can achieve basic proficiency in the application of IPT when closely supervised by a well-trained supervisor in 16 weeks of acute treatment of older adults with depression.

Our own research on family issues in late-life depression documented the presence of interpersonal stresses in the care of older adults with depression and the role of interpersonal factors on the course of the depression. Use of IPT to address interpersonal issues identified in that study seemed a logical clinical next step. Despite the large well-designed continuation/maintenance study of IPT in the treatment of late-life depression (Reynolds et al., 1999), the usefulness of IPC in the treatment of depressive symptoms in medically ill older adults (Mossey et al., 1996), and some pilot data on IPT in the acute treatment of late-life depression, the lack of a large, well-controlled study of acute IPT in the treatment of major depression in older adults is an empirical lacuna. Though others have commented, "Yet why expect IPT *not* to work with the elderly, as with other ages, in treating major depression?" (Weissman et al., 2000, p. 214), the critical IPT study in the treatment of acute depression in older adults remains to be conducted. Nonetheless, it is impressive that, in conjunction with antidepressant medication, the University of Pittsburgh researchers found excellent clinical outcomes in the acute and continuation treatment of older adults with recurrent depression—outcomes that did not differ from those of younger adults (Reynolds et al., 1999). In the maintenance phase of their study of depression in older adults, both antidepressant medication and minimal monthly IPT significantly reduced the likelihood of relapse—and the combination appeared to be the best.

In our clinical view, IPT is often the treatment of choice for older adults with major depression as well as adjustment disorder with depressive symptoms in which there is an interpersonally relevant problem. IPT has a well-defined structure but also a considerable latitude in how it can be implemented that builds on the skill and interpersonal sensitivity that many clinicians possess. It is compatible with contemporary use of antidepressant medication in the treatment of depression and facilitates collaboration with professionals prescribing that medication. IPT is consonant with the current emphasis in medicine and mental health on delivering treatments that are evidence-based. As such, it is managed care friendly yet has a patient-centered stance.

In the chapters that follow, we discuss the implementation of IPT with older adults with depression. Though our discussion of IPT mirrors the outline and principles originally articulated for younger adults, we emphasize clinical problems that often arise for older adults and discuss common issues in the implementation of IPT with this age group. Readers interested in using IPT in their clinical work should also read the *Comprehensive Guide to Interpersonal Psychotherapy* (Weissman et al., 2000) as it is the primary source for the implementation of IPT. As has been the case for us, we trust that those who choose to use IPT with older adults will find that it will enrich their psychotherapeutic work with older adults as well as improve clinical outcomes.

5

THE INITIAL SESSIONS

The therapist establishes the groundwork for interpersonal psycho-therapy (IPT) in the initial sessions. This critical phase of IPT establishes the basic frame for the therapy and begins to socialize the client into the language, concepts, and interpersonal focus of IPT. In our clinic, older clients have already had an initial evaluation before referral to IPT, so clinicians have in-hand basic information about the client's diagnosis, psychiatric history, medical problems and currently prescribed psychiatric and nonpsychiatric medications, brief social and occupational history, and discussion and education about acquired immune deficiency syndrome (AIDS). If an extensive evaluation is not done prior to the therapist's first contact with the client, this should be done on the initial visit. Some may find it surprising that AIDS is part of an initial discussion with older adults as it is often assumed that they are not at risk for AIDS. Although it is rare that older adults at our clinic present with AIDS, we find that some older adults engage in nonprotected sexual activity. In the case example that follows we demonstrate that AIDS is not unknown to older people. For those clients who have had an initial intake, we review the information with them in the first session to make sure it is correct and complete. We also find that reviewing this material provides us with our first opportunity to begin establishing the therapeutic relationship. If the older adult does not have an initial evaluation prior to commencing IPT, a thorough assessment should be completed as outlined in chapter 2 (this volume). Assessment of medical issues and cognitive functioning is especially important with this age group in light of increasing prevalence of health and cognitive problems. Written or verbal communications with the client's primary care physician may be helpful especially if there are complicated medical problems or questions about whether the onset of depression may be related to medical problems or prescribed medications. Nonphysician Medicare providers are, in fact, required, with the client's permission, to communicate with the client's physician. For those clients receiving psychiatric medications, collaboration with the individual prescribing the medications is important. Cognizance of and accommodations for possible sensory deficits (notably vision and hearing) are also important for older people.

DEAL WITH THE DEPRESSION

In the first session the focus is on depression (see Exhibit 5.1). We usually administer a psychiatric rating scale such as the HRSD in the first session (or no later than the second session), although other depression rating scales can of course be used. Use of a depression rating scale not only quickly focuses discussion on symptoms but also yields an objective index of the severity of depression against which future change in symptoms may be reviewed with the client. We find that older adults welcome quantification of symptoms. As many older adults have health problems, they are familiar with numerical summaries of health status. Some older adults are quite familiar with their cholesterol levels and blood pressure readings and see improvement in these indices as evidence of compliance with medical regimens and health. The meaning of the rating scale score is explained to the client (e.g., "according to your score, you have a moderately severe depression").

The therapist gives the depressive syndrome a name. Most clients we have seen in IPT have major depression and some have adjustment disorder with depressed or anxious mood or both. Occasionally major depression is concurrent with dysthymia. This combination is sometimes referred to as double depression (Keller & Shapiro, 1982). Although IPT continuation/maintenance research on older adults has focused on major depression, one study considered the usefulness of IPT with older adults in primary care with depressive symptoms (Mossey, Knott, Higgins, & Talerico, 1996). For clients with adjustment disorder, we follow the standard IPT protocol developed for those with MDD. We find that older clients rarely have a specific name for the depressive condition they are experiencing or they use more colloquial means of describing the depression (*nervous breakdown, depression, nerves, stress*). This is even the case for older adults who have had long histo-

EXHIBIT 5.1
Outline of Interpersonal Psychotherapy for Major Depression

I. The Initial Sessions
    A. Dealing With the Depression
        1. Review depressive symptoms.
        2. Give the syndrome a name.
        3. Explain depression as a medical illness; and explain the treatment.
        4. Give the patient the "sick role."
        5. Evaluate the need for medication.
    B. Relate Depression to Interpersonal Context
        1. Review current and past interpersonal relationships as they relate to current depressive symptoms. Determine with the patient the
            a. nature of interaction with significant persons;
            b. expectations of patient and significant persons from one another, and whether these were fulfilled;
            c. satisfying and unsatisfying aspects of the relationships;
            d. changes the patient wants in the relationships.
    C. Identification of Major Problem Areas
        1. Determine the problem area related to current depression and set the treatment goals.
        2. Determine which relationship or aspect of a relationship is related to the depression and what might change in it.
    D. Explain the IPT Concepts and Contract
        1. Outline your understanding of the problem.
        2. Agree on treatment goals, determining which problem area will be the focus.
        3. Describe procedures of IPT: "here and now" focus, need for patient to discuss important concerns; review of current interpersonal relations; discussion of practical aspects of treatment—length, frequency, times, fees, policy for missed appointments.

Note. From *Comprehensive Guide to Interpersonal Psychotherapy* (p. 22), by M. M. Weissman, J. C. Markowitz, and G. L. Klerman, 2000, New York: Basic Books. Copyright 2000 by Basic Books. Reprinted with permission.

ries of depression. One suspects that prior clinicians failed to provide a diagnostic label or mentioned it only once and never referred to it again. We find this situation surprising because many older adults can provide accurate labeling of medical conditions and some have actively sought out information about medical problems. We use *DSM–IV* language to describe the diagnosis and may open the *Diagnostic and Statistical Manual of Mental Disorders, Fourth Edition* (*DSM–IV*) and read characteristic symptoms to the client. Sometimes use of the *DSM–IV* to review symptoms is a powerful intervention in itself as older adults express surprise and relief that they are not the only person who is experiencing their difficulties and that experts well understand the nature of their symptoms. We might also give a brief summary of the frequency of depression in older adults and common risk-factors of depression among them.

Depression is characterized as a medical illness. Defining depression as a medical illness may be puzzling to some older adults who grew up in an era when psychiatric problems were characterized as moral failing, lack of will, or weakness. However, as most older adults have one or more medical problems, they are familiar with the medical paradigm and, with some explanation, most are accepting of it. For others, further explanation and discussion are useful. We find that a discussion of the mind–body connection makes sense especially when we point to the vegetative signs of major depression such as sleep and appetite changes as well as how depression makes it more difficult to function, as when they are physically ill. Treatments for depression, including medication and psychotherapy, are reviewed. We discuss ECT if the client has previously been treated with this modality or it has been recommended. Citing some of the clinical research noted in chapters 3 and 4 (this volume), we explain that psychotherapy alone or in combination with psychiatric medication has been found to significantly improve depressive symptoms in the majority of adults and share our own clinical experience in treating older adults with depression.

The client is given the "sick role." As noted earlier, the notion of the sick role derives from sociologists' observation that it is normative for medically ill individuals to have temporary respite from daily responsibilities until they are well (Klerman et al., 1984). Some older adults are puzzled as to why they are having difficulty functioning and blame themselves for "not trying harder" or being "lazy." These attributions may generate feelings of guilt or self-criticism. A review of problems in functioning and a restatement of the fact that difficulty in functioning is part and parcel of their medical illness may be helpful. Conveying one's own expectation that the older person will return to functioning once the depression has improved engenders hopefulness. The older client is encouraged to temporarily reduce or refrain from obligations that he or she is having difficulty fulfilling. Some novice IPT therapists wonder whether such a strategy will convey to the person that little is expected of him or her and make it less likely that the client will make active efforts to improve. As is seen later, the middle sessions focus on what the client can actually do to contend with problematic issues in a manner that acknowledges how difficult it may be to function yet encourages activities that improve the situation.

The therapist then evaluates the need for psychiatric medication. In our clinic any need for psychiatric medication has already been noted at the initial evaluation. When an evaluation has not taken place, those clinicians who can prescribe medications should make this assessment. Nonprescribing clinicians who feel the client could benefit from medication need to make a referral for a medication evaluation. Some older adults refuse to take psychiatric medications for fear that the medications are "addicting," because they "take too many medications already," or because they "should be able to handle this myself." For older adults with severe major depression where psychiatric medications have been strongly recommended, we devote more time to a discussion of medication and their reluctance to take it. We encourage the client in initial and later sessions to reconsider the decision not to take medications.

RELATE DEPRESSION TO THE INTERPERSONAL CONTEXT

Usually by the second session the therapist conducts an interpersonal inventory to get an overview of current and relevant past interpersonal relationships. We find that the series of questions in the IPT outline is a useful method for conducting this inquiry. Because the clinician usually has no more than one session to gather this information, it is important to be goal-directed in inquiry. The need for a time-limited review of interpersonal relations can be signaled to the older client by saying something such as "I'd like to get a general sense of the important people in your life. At this point we won't go into detail about those relationships, but talk for 5 or 10 minutes about each person you feel is important to you." We find that without making the time limit clear some older adults will go into considerable detail about each relationship in a way that makes it difficult to complete the interpersonal inventory in the allotted time. In light of the fact that older adults have a lifetime of interpersonal relationships, it is advisable to focus on current relationships but also discuss important, relevant past relationships that may have a bearing on current circumstances. The interpersonal inventory provides important information on existing interpersonally relevant problems (that will likely be the focus of therapy) and also gives a general sense of the client's interpersonal strengths and weaknesses. Some individuals have chronically problematic relationships to which they have adapted and see as normative, and which would not have been revealed early in treatment if the inventory had not been completed.

IDENTIFY MAJOR PROBLEM AREAS

Information gleaned through the interpersonal inventory and the client's informal account of the circumstances surrounding depression will yield important clues to the problem area or areas that will be the focus of treatment. We are especially interested in what was happening in the client's life just prior to the onset of depression. If the client has had prior episodes of depression we are also interested in ascertaining possible psychosocial precipitants of those episodes. Apparent precipitants may reveal specific domains of interpersonal events in which the client is vulnerable to depression. For example, an older client may have had the onset of depression when previously dealing with health issues or disputes with significant others. For some clients there is no apparent precipitant, but the onset of depression created or exacerbated existing conflicts with a significant other. In initial sessions the client occasionally cannot identify any interpersonally relevant event, in which case IPT may not be the best paradigm for treatment. We have found clinically that clients with prominent anxiety or pronounced maladaptive cognitions are better treated with cognitive–behavioral therapy (discussed in chap. 2, this volume), which has a good track record in the treatment of late-life depression. With identification of the interpersonal problem area, the therapist works with the client to establish treatment goals. One treatment goal that we set with all clients is a significant reduction in depressive symptoms. Other goals are set on the basis of the identified problem area and mirror goals articulated for each of those areas. For example, a goal for an older adult with a dispute might be to "better understand and deal with difficulties in the relationship with your husband." A goal for those with grief could be to "come to terms with the loss of your wife and move on in your life." A goal for a client with role transition could be to "deal with the change in your life since your husband was diagnosed with Alzheimer's disease and figure out how to better manage the many responsibilities you now have for his care." For an older adult with interpersonal deficits, the goal might be to "figure out a way to develop new friendships so that you feel less isolated."

Some clients have two problem areas that will be the focus of treatment. One of the problem areas is typically given greater emphasis in the therapy on the basis of its relationship to the onset of depression and emotional salience to the client. In view of the time-limited nature of IPT in the acute treatment of depression, no more than two areas can be accommodated in the 16-week therapy. We often find that the secondary problem area germinates from the first. For example, depression following role transition or grief may generate an interpersonal dispute with a significant other because of the interpersonal tensions often found among persons with depression and their primary relationships.

EXPLAIN THE IPT CONCEPTS AND CONTRACT

In the third and final meeting of the initial sessions, the therapist provides an interpersonal formulation to the client. The clinician reviews and restates the fact that the client has a medical illness, using the name of the depressive syndrome; explains his or her understanding of the interpersonally relevant event that appeared to precipitate the depression and any interpersonal problems that were seeded by the depression; and identifies the problem area or areas that will be the focus of treatment and associated treatment goals. After giving this formulation to the client, we invite his or her input to make sure "that I correctly understand things." Most older people concur with the therapist's summary statement and some express delight that the therapist has correctly and succinctly characterized their problems. The client occasionally disagrees with one or more aspects of the formulation. In this case, further discussion is required so that there is at least tentative concurrence on treatment goals. Some older adults may not initially concur because they are skeptical that a 16-week treatment could be helpful or are doubtful that the problematic issue could actually be resolved through psychotherapy. Some older adults have had experience in prior psychotherapy such as extended psychoanalysis or psychodynamic psychotherapy and wonder whether these treatments might be better than IPT. The client is given the option to pursue other psychotherapeutic options if he or she feels strongly about it. Our experience is that almost all of the older adults we have treated who have reservations are willing to give IPT a try.

In the third session the therapist concludes with a description of the structure of IPT. The therapist may offer a simple explanation that research has found IPT to be useful in most cases, stating that he or she is hopeful about the client's prognosis. Also provided is an explanation that IPT generally focuses on things that are going on in the present although there can be discussion of past life events that seem relevant to current problems. The clinician emphasizes that it is important for the client to discuss things that are of concern. The therapist also reviews the 16-week time frame of the therapy, the fact that there will be weekly meetings, and the established time and date of the meetings. Barring illness, inclement weather, or unexpected life events, it is anticipated that the client will attend weekly sessions. Some older adults unfamiliar with psychotherapy are occasionally surprised that psychotherapy will extend beyond a few sessions because their experience with medical care providers is only occasional appointments.

In summary, in the initial sessions the therapist conveys that he or she understands the client's problems, has a plan for addressing them, and is hopeful that treatment will be useful. With this explanation some older adults begin to evidence some improvement as they begin to feel more hopeful that things can improve.

CASE EXAMPLES

In the remainder of this chapter we provide four case examples of initial sessions with older clients for whom the primary problem areas are grief, interpersonal role disputes, role transition, and interpersonal deficits, respectively. The cases are from our clinical work with older adults. First and last names used in the clinical examples are fictitious. We have changed several aspects of each case or used composites of cases to protect the confidentiality of these individuals while conveying the substance of each case. We trust that the case examples are useful in illustrating the goals, strategies, and techniques of IPT with older adults. So the reader can have a sense of continuity of these cases from beginning to end, each case is discussed further in a following chapter that is relevant to the primary problem area of the client. We also use one additional case to illustrate each of the primary problem areas.

Grief: The Case of Gloria Johnson

Mrs. Johnson, a 69-year-old, Protestant, Caucasian, married woman was referred to the therapist after an initial evaluation by a clinic staff member who provided a diagnosis of major depression, single episode, mild. She had a medical diagnosis of hypertension and was taking an antihypertensive medication. There was no evidence of cognitive impairment. She was referred for psychotherapy because of difficulty in coming to terms with the death of her brother and sister-in-law who had died within a short time of each other. Since their deaths over a year ago, she had become increasingly depressed, had less interest in seeing friends, and found daily responsibilities an increasing burden. In the first session the HRSD was administered and she had a score of 18 (i.e., *moderate depression*). Symptoms were discussed with her and an explanation of major depression, including its characterization as a medical illness, was provided. She was familiar with the concept of major depression because her sister-in-law had been treated for it while she was dying and she had done some reading on the topic. The therapist told Mrs. Johnson that her difficulties with functioning were tied to major depression, that these were typical of major depression, and that in the short run she might want to limit social involvement so they felt less burdensome as well as consider the possibility of hiring someone to help her with housework. Antidepressant medication had been recommended by the psychiatrist but Mrs. Johnson said that she was not interested in taking it at this time as she was hopeful that psychotherapy would alleviate symptoms. The therapist explained the usefulness of medication and that it should be especially helpful in reducing somatic symptoms of depression. She said that if she did not show improvement she would reconsider her decision.

The therapist inquired about the circumstances of her brother and sister-in-law's deaths. She said that they had died after "long illnesses" but was vague in describing what illnesses they had. "They just grew weaker and weaker and had problems fighting off illness." As the therapist continued to inquire about their medical problems, Mrs. Johnson grew more quiet and began to sob. "It's been a nightmare. Just a nightmare. I can't believe this happened. Not to me, not to them." Slowly she explained that her brother had a series of unexplained illnesses for which physicians could not find a cause. Then her sister began to grow weak and eventually contracted pneumonia. "How can I tell you this? They both had AIDS." She said that she couldn't understand how they had contracted AIDS. "I cared for them both. First my brother died, then my sister-in-law. How could I tell my friends what was going on? I just couldn't. Of course I told my husband but he was as horrified and embarrassed as I was."

In the next session the therapist conducted the interpersonal inventory. The inventory revealed that during her brother and sister-in-law's illness things grew more tense with her husband and that when she began to get depressed they had increasing conflict. She found that her husband was less and less available to support her as she was grieving the loss of her relatives. "I couldn't talk to my friends and eventually I didn't feel I could talk to him about this AIDS nightmare." She said that she and her husband had a reasonably good marriage but felt they were mismatched in temperament and interests. She wished her relationship with her husband would be less conflictual. She had a son and daughter with whom she had a good relationship and whom she eventually told the cause of her brother and sister-in-law's deaths. Although they were supportive, they both lived in another part of the country and she felt their absence. She had a history of an active and satisfying social life with friends and civic organizations but she said that having to "lie" about the cause of her relatives' deaths made her feel alienated from her friends and that since the onset of her depression about 6 months ago, she saw less of her friends.

The identified primary problem area was grief with a secondary problem area being interpersonal role disputes with her husband. Grief was identified as the primary problem area because it appeared to be the chief precipitant of the major depression and she felt it was the most important issue for her. Exacerbation of difficulties with her husband was consistent with research that has found that depression can seed interpersonal problems (Joiner, 2000). Goals of treatment were discussed with Mrs. Johnson, including resolution of the major depression, coming to terms with the deaths of her brother and sister-in-law, and improvement in the relationship with her husband. She felt that having an opportunity to talk honestly about her relatives' deaths would be beneficial and that reduction in conflict with her husband would make her life easier.

In the third session the therapist presented his understanding of her difficulties. "You are experiencing a major depression, which is a medical illness that, among other things, has made it much more difficult for you to socialize and to carry on daily responsibilities. Your depression followed the illness and deaths of your brother and sister-in-law, which was made especially difficult because you did not feel you could be honest with your friends and others about the fact they had AIDS. You have strong and complicated feelings about this that you have not been able to adequately sort out. Although your relationship with your husband has never been an ideal one, the stresses of your relatives' illnesses and the onset of your own psychiatric illness have resulted in conflict with your husband so that now you don't feel that you even have him to lean on. Do I understand things correctly?" Mrs. Johnson said yes but emphasized that the most important issue to contend with was the deaths of her relatives. She felt that if she was more resolved about this issue, things would likely improve with her husband but agreed that "my marriage needs some work."

The therapist explained the basic parameters of the IPT treatment. "IPT is a psychotherapy that was developed to help with the type of concerns that you have. Research and my own clinical experience indicate that the majority of people treated with IPT show significant improvement by the end of treatment. We will focus on issues that are going on in your life now and will also discuss the difficult circumstances surrounding your brother and sister-in-law's deaths. This appointment time seems to work for you and we will plan to get together each week for a total of 16 weeks. I encourage you to be candid and open with me about issues of concern as you feel that you haven't been able to do that with other people." The therapist again raised the option of antidepressant medication, which Mrs. Johnson said she would think about.

Interpersonal Role Disputes: The Case of Mary Ryan

Mrs. Ryan, a 79-year-old, widowed, Catholic woman, was referred for psychotherapy because of an estranged relationship with her older sister and a diagnosis of major depressive disorder, recurrent, moderate. She had had arthritis for several years and took anti-inflammatory medication to relieve discomfort, but generally characterized herself as being in good health. She had no evidence of cognitive impairment. Mrs. Ryan was somewhat puzzled by the referral for psychotherapy because she had gone to the doctor to get "something for my nerves." She said that she had found it increasingly difficult to spend time by herself because when she was alone she keep thinking about problems with her sister. "Sometimes I just run out of the house to get away from myself." She said that her nerves had grown worse in the past 6 months and at the same time she had problems with sleeping and was losing weight. She saw her internist who could find no medical basis for these symptoms and referred her to our psychiatric clinic.

Her score on the HRSD was 22, which indicated *significant depression*. Mrs. Ryan did not think of herself as depressed but rather as "nervous." And though she had a moderate degree of anxiety, her symptom picture fit a classical description of major depression. The therapist went through the list of symptoms associated with major depression from the *DSM–IV* and after reading each symptom, he asked, "Have you had problems with that?" She was surprised and even a little amused that "that book you're reading from could have been written about me." She reluctantly accepted the notion that she was experiencing a depression, albeit with a fair amount of anxiety. The therapist went into some detail about the nature of depression as a medical illness that can make it as difficult to function as can conditions such as heart disease or cancer. She recalled that she had felt the same way after her husband had died several years ago. Treatments for major depression were explained but she expressed disbelief that "just talking to somebody" could help a situation as difficult as she was experiencing with her sister. Mrs. Ryan said that she had to push herself to socialize, which was made all the more difficult because she and her estranged sister belonged to the same church social clubs. The therapist told her that it made perfect sense that it was difficult to do things because "as the book explained" major depression makes it much harder to get through the day. A psychiatrist had prescribed an SSRI antidepressant as well as a short course of a benzodiazepine for anxiety. She welcomed taking psychiatric medications.

The interpersonal inventory started with her sister. She and her sister had been close throughout their lives. They were part of a large extended family that gathered regularly. She and her sister used to see each other several times a week and talk regularly on the phone. As noted, they also belonged to several social organizations where they had a common set of friends and activities. She said that her sister was always "pushy," "kept me under her thumb," and "continued to treat me as a little sister." She said that until recent years she had accepted this subordinate position but I "began to answer back to my sister, which she didn't like." Things came to a head in the prior year when she and her sister took a tour of Ireland. During the trip her sister twisted her ankle and insisted that Mrs. Ryan return home with her. Mrs. Ryan did not feel that her sister's injury was severe enough to return home and refused. They continued on the trip, during which time she helped her sister but "after that she never forgave me." On their return home her sister complained to family members that she had been abandoned by Mrs. Ryan, would barely speak to her at social club meetings, and refused to acknowledge her at family gatherings. "I tried to talk to her but it always ended up in a fight." In the past 4 to 5 months, as she grew hopeless of a rapprochement with her sister, symptoms of major depression developed.

Other relationships were reviewed. She said that she had had a generally satisfactory relationship with her now deceased husband. After his death she said she struggled with having to take over household responsibilities. She said that she felt overwhelmed and became depressed. She recovered from the depression without treatment and, much to her surprise, learned that she was more independent and resourceful than she had previously believed. She had three daughters, all of whom lived in her vicinity and with whom she had generally good relationships. In addition, she had numerous brothers and sisters, with all of whom she had congenial relations. Over the years she had a high level of social involvement, which she enjoyed.

In the third session, relevant issues were reviewed with her. "As we discussed, you have a major depression, which is a medical illness that has made it much more difficult for you to function. As often happens with major depression, you also have quite of bit of anxiety, which you call *nerves*. As the depression improves you will feel not only less depressed but also less anxious. To me it seems fairly clear that the onset of your illness followed the dispute with your sister over what happened in Ireland. Although you've tried to make things better with your sister, your efforts seem to you to have only made things worse. I think we can set some goals for the psychotherapy. At the end of treatment one goal would be that you feel much less depressed. Another goal would be for you to have made efforts to improve your relationship with your sister." Mrs. Ryan said that it was hard to believe that things could improve because her sister was so stubborn, and she again recounted that her efforts to "make up" with her sister had been rebuffed. She said that she would be satisfied if her sister would treat her more politely at church social meetings and family gatherings. She said that family members had expressed dismay and disappointment with their behavior with each other and thought it was "ridiculous" that at their age they were engaging in a feud. The session concluded with a discussion of IPT as a treatment modality, its focus on the present, the importance of raising issues of concern with the therapist, and frequency of meetings. She was also reminded that the duration of the treatment would be 16 weeks. "I'll give it a try. What else can I do?" remarked Mrs. Ryan.

Role Transition: The Case of May Barton

May Barton was a 74-year-old, married, Caucasian woman, who was referred for psychotherapy after an initial evaluation by clinic staff. She was diagnosed with major depressive disorder, recurrent, mild. She had osteoporosis, which had worsened in recent years and for which she took medication along with a vitamin regimen that she believed would improve the condition. She felt that the osteoporosis made it more difficult for her to do housework and somewhat limited her ambulation. Although she had complained of memory problems, there was no evidence of significant cognitive impairment. Several years ago she had been treated for what appeared to have been a severe episode of major depression that had lasted 2 or 3 years. She had been prescribed a variety of antidepressant medications that did not seem to help. She subsequently had a course of psychotherapy, after which the depression remitted. The most recent episode of depression had lasted 4 months. It is likely she also had had another episode of major depression in earlier life.

In the first session the clinician reviewed information from the initial evaluation and the HRSD was administered. She had a score of 14, which indicated *mild* to *moderate depression*. Although Mrs. Barton was unfamiliar with the term *major depression*, she readily accepted the explanation that depression was an illness. "When I was depressed before, I realized I was in big trouble. I could hardly get out of bed or even clean up the kitchen. I didn't want to see anyone and everyone kept asking me what was wrong. I said that I didn't know." She said that there was no apparent precipitant of the depression. She made it clear that her current depressive problems were not as severe as they were in the prior episode. "I'm scared though. I don't want to end up like that again." Mrs. Barton understood that psychiatric medication and psychotherapy were usual treatments for depression. She was emphatic, however: "I will not take antidepressant medication. They didn't work for me before and made me into a zombie." It appeared that Mrs. Barton's internist had previously prescribed tricyclic antidepressant medications, including several that are well known to have anticholinergic side effects including constipation, blurry vision, dry mouth, and orthostatic hypotension. The therapist explained that newer medications had many fewer side effects and that most older adults found them much easier to take than medications she had previously taken. "I'm sorry, but I'm not taking antidepressant medication."

Mrs. Barton's chief complaint was that it was increasingly difficult to care for her husband. "It's so hard to get through the day." The therapist explained that major depression made it more difficult to function, a notion that she readily accepted. She said that osteoporosis made it more challenging to take care of home responsibilities but the biggest problem was knowing how to deal with her husband, who had grown increasingly forgetful and disoriented since his recent strokes. "I don't know what to do with him. Sometimes I just lose it."

In the second session the therapist conducted the interpersonal inventory. She said that she had had a "good marriage" of over 50 years to her husband, Peter, who was a retired fireman. Although in later years her husband developed diabetes, it was reasonably well controlled with medication and diet. "And then came the stroke. About 3 years ago he had a stroke. It left him weak on one side and he needed a walker for a while. He improved a lot from physical therapy though. The therapist pushed him very hard to do better and he did." Nonetheless she had to take on many more household responsibilities because of her husband's disability. This was made more difficult because of osteoporosis but she felt she managed. It was notable that Mrs. Barton did not experience significant symptoms of depression that time.

"And then came the second and third strokes about 6 months ago. We were so happy that he lived through those but after that he just wasn't the same. I'd tell him something and he'd forget. I'd ask him why he didn't shave and he'd say 'I did,' but he hadn't and then I'd get mad at him. He just sits in front of the TV all day and I tell him he needs to do something. He says 'sure' and then just continues watching TV. I get so upset with him and then feel bad about doing that." It seemed apparent to the therapist that Mrs. Barton's husband had dementia and he commented that it was common for family members caring for persons with dementia to feel frustrated and upset. "Dementia? Doctor, my husband is not a case from a textbook." The therapist asked to what she attributed her husband's change in behavior. She said it was his recent strokes and acknowledged that medical staff had mentioned the word *dementia*. They had even given her a brochure on dementia but she did not read it. When asked why she didn't read it, she replied, "I know about those things." She said, however, that she'd like to learn how to better deal with her husband now that his condition had grown worse.

Other relationships were reviewed. She seemed to have reasonably good relationships with family members and friends while growing up. She expressed delight in raising her daughter who was now married and lived in another state. They had a good relationship, speaking regularly on the phone, but she was sad that her daughter did not live closer. Nonetheless, she felt she could rely on her daughter and in an emergency her daughter would help. She described a history of relationships with a small number of friends, most of whom she had known since childhood. When asked about other social involvements she described herself as "not a joiner" and said that she didn't feel comfortable in groups "like the kind you'd find at church. My husband liked clubs and organizations." When asked about other important relationships, she paused and said, "There's a woman in our home now who helps my husband. That hasn't been so easy." She explained that since her husband's latest strokes, a home health care aide assisted him every day and that she found the presence of the aide uncomfortable. "She seems lazy and I don't know how to get her to do what is needed. Maybe it's culture or something. She's from Russia and it's hard to understand her because of her accent. Do you know she's unmarried and has a child?"

In the third session the therapist gave an interpersonal formulation to Mrs. Barton. "As we've discussed, you have major depression, which, although it is not as severe as the one you experienced several years ago, is nonetheless a milder form of the illness you've experienced. The depression followed Peter's most recent strokes. You feel like you don't know how to handle things now—especially since your husband has had memory problems." (At this point the therapist was mindful of Mrs. Barton's sensitivity to the use of the word *dementia* and felt that further discussion of the nature of this condition would wait until the therapeutic relationship was better developed.) "You have what we would call in this psychotherapy a *role transition*. That is, you've moved from being a caregiver to someone with physical health problems to a caregiver to someone with physical disabilities as well as memory problems. This has presented you with the challenge of trying to figure out how to handle this new change in your husband's behavior." Mrs. Barton said this made sense to her. "In addition, you now have a home health aide in your home who is different from you. You also face the fact that you are now an employer and are not quite sure how to get the aide to do what you expect of her." Mrs. Barton reminded the therapist that she had always been a homemaker and never had experience in the workplace.

"I think there are two major goals for psychotherapy. The first goal is that you will be less depressed by the end of therapy. The second goal is that you will be more capable in handling the new problems you're dealing with in care of your husband including management of the home health aide. Do these seem like reasonable goals to you?" She said that this made sense to her but reiterated that she would not take antidepressant medication. "I understand that you feel strongly about that issue. I feel reasonably confident that by the end of therapy you will be less depressed and in a better position to handle things." Finally, the therapist reviewed the time frame of IPT, the focus on current problems, the need for Mrs. Barton to share any concerns she had about the therapy, and planned meeting times.

Interpersonal Deficits: The Case of Rachel Greenberg

Rachel Greenberg was a 62-year-old, unmarried, unemployed, Jewish woman who was diagnosed by clinic staff with major depression, single episode, severe. She had a history of scoliosis of the spine, cataracts, and hearing loss. She did not take any medications for her health conditions. She evidenced no cognitive impairment. She had been referred to our clinic by her primary care physician who had started her on an antidepressant medication, which initially did not seem to improve depressive symptoms. On initial meeting, curvature of her spine was apparent despite the fact that the client insisted on wearing a winter coat throughout the session. In the initial meeting she seemed nervous and made little eye contact. She said that her mother had died 6 months previously after an extended illness. Given her apparent discomfort, the therapist decided to wait until the second session to administer the HRSD. The circumstances of her mother's illness were discussed and the client explained that her mother had an increasing number of medical problems and then developed dementia. Ms. Greenberg quit her job as an office worker to care for her mother and eventually hired a home health aide to assist her. She felt that inattention by the aide led to a fall that her mother experienced, which led to a hospitalization. Shortly thereafter her mother died of complications of the fall. Ms. Greenberg was at times tearful in discussing care for her mother. "While she was sick I realized that I was getting older too. Who would care for me if I got sick?" Ms. Greenberg seemed to be more relaxed by the end of the session and said that it was helpful to talk to somebody who seemed to care.

In the second session the therapist reviewed depressive symptoms based on the initial evaluation report and also by administering the HRSD, on which Ms. Greenberg got a score of 27, indicating *significant depression*. The client said that though she had had periods in her life in which she felt "discouraged" and "down," she had never felt this way before. The therapist explained, "You have a major depression, which is different than the normal ups and downs that we all experience. The changes you've seen in recent months—depressed mood, anxiety, problems with sleeping, weight gain, difficulty doing things, discouragement, hopelessness—these are part of the medical illness that you are now experiencing." The therapist described the usefulness of psychotherapy and antidepressant medication in the treatment of depression. Ms. Greenberg said that she was discouraged that the antidepressant medication did not seem to help. As Ms. Greenberg said that she had been taking antidepressant medication for only a month, the therapist explained that sometimes it may take a bit longer for medication to work. Even if the current medication she was taking didn't help, there were many different antidepressant medications and the psychiatrist prescribing the medication might consider another one in the future.

In reviewing her functioning, it became apparent that Ms. Greenberg had minimal responsibilities or involvement in her life. Nonetheless, she found it difficult to keep her home maintained as she had previously. She was encouraged to temporarily lower her expectations about how clean her home should be until she was feeling better. "*If* I feel better," she corrected the therapist. "*When* you feel better," replied the therapist. "I think I'm more hopeful about things than you are. But that makes sense because you're depressed and depressed people usually see the glass half empty. This is a very treatable illness."

The interpersonal inventory was begun toward the end of the second session and continued into the third session. Ms. Greenberg said that she had never married. The therapist was attentive to the possibility that Ms. Greenberg had had prior relationships with women and framed questions in a way that did not prejudge her sexual orientation. "Even though you've never married have there been people in your life with whom you had an intimate relationship?" She said that she had once kissed a boy when she was younger but other than that she had never been physical with anyone. It appeared that Ms. Greenberg had no history of sexual or intimate relations.

"My mother was my life." She had always lived with and been close to her mother. She said that generally they had had a good relationship although she expressed regret that she had not been more patient with her mother during the last years of her illness. "She was always so encouraging to me. She'd offer me suggestions on how to get to know people and get along with them but people were always hard for me." A discussion of earlier-life relations revealed a paucity of connections with other people starting in high school. "In high school my problem became pretty obvious to other kids." The therapist inquired as to what problem she was referring. She answered, "You know," and pointed to her back. "The scoliosis?" "Yes, the scoliosis." She gave an account of endless taunts from peers during high school because of the deformity caused by scoliosis. She said that peers called her cruel names and that she had been pushed down on the ground by girls who said she was ugly, and recounted an incident when a boy spit in her face. "All I wanted to do was to get away from people and be with my mother." She entered the workforce as a young woman and appeared to have functioned well in various clerical capacities but kept her distance socially from coworkers. She related incidents from her work life in which coworkers had said things to her that she perceived as critical of her appearance and shyness.

Nonetheless, she had relationships with a circle of relatives whom she saw at regular family gatherings and with whom she felt comfortable. The problem she faced now was that many of these relatives were dead, were ill, had moved away, or were involved primarily with their own children and grandchildren. She had one brother with whom she had a good relationship. Her brother was married to a woman she did not like and who she felt at times was disrespectful of her. "My sister-in-law once told me I was pathetic."

Since her mother's death she relied more and more on her brother for practical help and emotional support yet she felt his wife discouraged contact with her.

Ms. Greenberg explained her dilemma. "My life was my mother. Now I have no life. I know that I have shied away from people and that wasn't good. But now I know that I need to have some people in my life. I just don't feel comfortable with people. I'm very shy and think that other people won't like me. I worry about who will take care of me when I'm old. I just feel so depressed when I think about this and don't know what to do."

During the third session the therapist offered his interpersonal formulation that mirrored the information that Ms. Greenberg had shared. "The death of your mother marked a very big change in your life. You've had to deal with her loss but, more important, it seems you're confronting the reality that you don't have that many people in your world and you'd like more. On the basis of what you told me about your high school years, it makes good sense to me that you would be wary of other people. You were harassed and treated cruelly by your peers and that was terrible to go through. You adapted to things the best way you could but with the passing of your mother you face the challenge of establishing other relationships. This growing awareness was followed by the major depressive illness which makes it all the more difficult for you to take the steps you want to include more people in your world. It sounds like you'd also like to strengthen the ties to your brother but this is hard because you don't like his wife and believe she doesn't like you. Do I understand things correctly?" Ms. Greenberg said that this made sense to her.

"So, one important goal of this interpersonal psychotherapy will include significantly reducing the symptoms associated with your depressive illness. As I indicated, these symptoms make it very difficult to function. I will be in contact with your doctor from time to time to see if she wants to make any changes in your medication. The second goal is to help you to try to increase the number of people in your world, including bettering your relationship with your brother. I know this will be difficult but I am hopeful." The particulars of the therapy were reviewed with Ms. Greenberg, including its duration, focus on the present, importance of discussing issues of concern, and appointment times. Ms. Greenberg expressed appreciation for the therapist's understanding and comforting words.

6

GRIEF

Most older women experience widowhood and are almost three times as likely to be widowed as are men. Older women spend about 14 years of life as widows compared with 7 years for men. Two fifths of older people experience the death of a sibling. In later life some contend with the death of long-lived parents or adult children. With advancing years more and more friends, former coworkers, and acquaintances die (Gallagher-Thompson & Thompson, 1996; Moss, Moss, & Hansson, 2001). We have met some very old people who have literally outlived everyone important in their lives.

Bereavement is a natural response to loss of loved ones (Bonanno & Kaltman, 2001). The constellation of emotional, physical, and cognitive responses to the death of a significant other—called grief or bereavement—is the norm. For those who have lost a spouse, acute emotional distress is most pronounced in the 2 to 6 months following death. Although a set number of stages of grieving or a firm timetable by which to judge "normal" bereavement have not been found, most older adults demonstrate considerable emotional recovery 1 year after the death of a spouse. Feelings of loss may persist indefinitely for some if not most (Gallagher-Thompson & Thompson, 1996; Hanson & Hayslip, 2000).

However, some older adults have considerable difficulties with bereavement. Although researchers debate where to draw the line between normal grief and complicated grief, some studies suggest that 1 year or more after spousal loss, 15% of widows meet criteria for major depression (Zisook & Shuchter, 1991) or have a severe or chronic grief reaction (Bonanno & Kaltman, 2001). Individuals with especially disabling, intense, or prolonged distress associated with bereavement—notably those with symptoms consistent with major depression—are likely candidates for pharmacological and psychotherapeutic intervention. Some argue that even older adults experiencing emotional distress typical of normal bereavement may benefit from antidepressant medication.

Several factors are associated with more intense or complicated grief. It is interesting that older adults adapt better to loss of spouse than do younger persons. Older men have a greater increased risk of death following the death of spouse than do older women. Likely reasons for this increased risk include loss of the wife's role in facilitation of social relationships and health-promoting behaviors.

Bereavement is more likely to be complicated when the loved one died of a stigmatizing illness such as AIDS or died from suicide. Presence of clinically significant symptoms within the first 2 months of a spouse's death is associated with poorer outcome. Availability of social support is tied to a better course of bereavement. Combinations of the above factors may increase the likelihood of prolonged bereavement and risk for a major depression (Gallagher-Thompson & Thompson, 1996). We know little about the impact of multiple personal losses on risk for complicated bereavement.

Recent work by Bonanno and colleagues (Bonanno & Kaltman, 2001) has challenged the assumption that successful recovery from interpersonal loss necessarily requires the mental or emotional working-through of the loss. They suggest that some individuals who show minimal affective expression about as well as minimal cognitive focus on the deceased evidence a successful bereavement. Using an adult development and aging perspective, Hanson and Hayslip (2000, p. 351) wondered whether individuals with a more complex sense of self adapt better to widowhood. "Individuals with a potentially more complex self-concept, containing a greater variety of current and possible selves are less threatened by the loss of one of their important identities (e.g., spouse)."

IPT TREATMENT OF GRIEF

Most older adults with complicated grief are contending with the loss of a spouse. Some get stuck in the grieving process because long-standing marital problems and their attendant ambivalent feelings toward the spouse psychologically complicate the bereavement process. Others have been long-time caregivers to a spouse with physical or cognitive disease, or both. Older adults who have had a very dependent relationship on the deceased spouse

I. Intermediate Sessions—The Problem Areas
  A. Grief
    1. Goals
      a. Facilitate the mourning process.
      b. Help the patient reestablish interest and relationships to substitute for what has been lost.
    2. Strategies
      a. Review depressive symptoms.
      b. Relate symptom onset to death of significant other.
      c. Reconstruct the patient's relationship with the deceased.
      d. Describe the sequence and consequences of events just prior to, during, and after the death.
      e. Explore associated feelings (negative as well as positive).
      f. Consider possible ways of becoming involved with others.

Note. From *Comprehensive Guide to Interpersonal Psychotherapy* (pp. 22–23), by M. M. Weissman, J. C. Markowitz, and G. L. Klerman, 2000, New York: Basic Books. Copyright 2000 by Basic Books. Reprinted with permission.

may not be able to come to terms with that reality or the challenges of establishing a new life structure. Family and friends sometimes criticize an older adult who needs an extended period of bereavement and refuse to discuss the deceased, thus cutting off the older adult from needed opportunities to process the loss. Some older clients are grieving the recent loss or remote loss of an adult child or grandchild. An older woman with serious depression recently came to our clinic because she was preoccupied with and unable to accept the death of her granddaughter who was killed by an automobile. Sibling death can be especially painful and complicated for older adults if the relationship was very close or, conversely, if a rupture in the relationship in earlier years was not mended before death.

GOALS AND STRATEGIES IN THE IPT TREATMENT OF GRIEF

As can been seen from the outline (see Exhibit 6.1), there are two straightforward goals in the interpersonal psychotherapy (IPT) treatment of grief: Facilitate the mourning process and help the patient reestablish interest and relationships to substitute for what has been lost. In the beginning of the intermediate sessions, the therapist's focus is on facilitation of mourning. By progressing in this area, the client begins to establish a new life structure. Usually the client is also less depressed halfway through therapy, which makes an increase in social involvement and activities easier. Until the very end of therapy, however, the mourning process is often intermingled with establishing a new life structure.

Strategy 2a: Review depressive symptoms. Throughout psychotherapy the therapist reviews the presence and severity of depression and associated symptoms. Conceptually disentangling symptoms of a major depression from normal symptoms of grief is a challenge because they overlap. Sometimes the therapist can say, "In addition to the feelings of grief that you are experiencing, you're also contending with a major depression, which makes it even more difficult for you to face the reality of the loss of your spouse."

Strategy 2b: Relate symptom onset to death of significant other. The connection between the death of a significant other and the onset of depression should have been reviewed by the therapist in the initial sessions. This connection bears repeating to the client by the therapist during the middle phases of treatment. Sometimes older clients are so depressed that they lose sight of the fact that there is a real-life reason for the way they feel. If depression has a cause (vs. the experience of depression as coming from somewhere for some reason and with little hope of going away), it can be coped with in a way that reduces depressive symptoms. Something that has a cause can have a cure.

Strategy 2c: Reconstruct the patient's relationship with the deceased. Although the primary focus of IPT is in the here and now, in the treatment of grief a fair amount of time will be devoted to the past relationship with the deceased person. In the initial sessions the therapist will gain an overview of the relationship the older client had with the deceased. The way in which the deceased is described may give some hint of where the grieving process may be stuck. Although grieving persons tend to characterize the deceased in ways that minimize less-than-favorable characteristics, pronounced minimization may suggest the need for a careful inquiry about problems in the relationship. Evasiveness about important details of the relationship may signal that the older person is having problems acknowledging feelings or concerns that, when discussed, could facilitate the grief process. IPT's specific techniques of exploration, encouragement of affect, and clarification will be especially helpful. (See chap. 3, this volume, for a discussion of these techniques.) Asking detailed questions is very useful to clarify relationship issues. Details help to move the older person beyond socially conventional scripts about the relationship, provide a clearer sense of past or current events, and elicit emotions. Some older persons repeat what they feel should be said about a spouse because they fear social embarrassment over revelation of the more complex reality of the relationship. Other older adults believe that a frank discussion of problems in a close relationship betrays family confidences to an outsider—even if that individual is a mental health professional. As noted in chapter 4, an older person's "life story" (McAdams, 1995), existing "life span construct" (Whitbourne, 1987), or projection of future self (Markus & Nurius, 1986) includes the deceased spouse and is a way of making sense of the world. Some people hold on to these stories or constructs in ways that do not accommodate past or current realities. Psychotherapy encourages a more honest reckoning with what is, has been, and likely will be. We often find that persons with complicated bereavement have ambivalent feelings toward the deceased that make it more difficult to grieve and move on.

Strategy 2d: Describe the sequence and consequences of events just prior to, during, and after the death. Some have characterized grief as a variant of posttraumatic stress (Schut, Stroebe, de Keijser, & van den Bout, 1997). Indeed, during the short or prolonged process of the death of a loved one, many older adults have witnessed very troubling things. Serious illness brings family members into the world of the hospital or nursing home where family members will see not only the fragility of their loved one but also that of others. Older clients have described the horror of invasive medical procedures, encounters with less-than-caring medical staff, postsurgical wounds, urinary and fecal incontinence, delirious behavior, hallucinations, and the many other faces of physical deterioration. Simply from an existential perspective, serious health problems leading to death confront an individual with the starkness of human frailty and the inevitability of death. With whom do you speak about these things? Family are sometimes reluctant to hear these accounts because they elicit painful emotions. Or, the family member with whom life's most poignant experiences have been shared is the person who is dying. Older clients tell us that friends and acquaintances are often reluctant to hear a full account of the painful end because they may have already experienced spousal loss or fear it. Thus some older adults have no one to whom they can turn.

We often find that giving the older client the opportunity to speak, in detail, about the circumstances surrounding the loved one's death is important. As mentioned earlier, the therapist may be the only person who welcomes the discussion. Therefore, the therapist needs to signal to the older client that it is okay to talk about the dying process—and signal this by gently but matter-of-factly asking specific questions. "What did your husband look like while he was dying?" "Did he seem to be in pain? How did you know that?" "How did you feel when you had to change his colostomy bag?" "Were you there the moment that she died?" The process of making funeral arrangements can also elicit important and affectively laden recollections that, on their telling, can be healing.

Strategy 2e: Explore associated feelings (negative as well as positive). This strategy is integrated during reconstruction of the relationship with the deceased and circumstances surrounding dying, and in review of options for reconstituting a new life to substitute for what has been lost. For those who have difficulty acknowledging less satisfactory aspects of the relationship with the deceased, it may be helpful to suggest that "All relationships have problems in them. What were some of the problems you and your spouse dealt with?" "What times were most stressful in your relationship?" "Were there things that you would have done differently?" In an accounting of the dying process, the client may be reluctant to admit to feelings of relief at the time of the relative's death. The therapist can encourage discussion of this by making comments such as "Some wives feel some relief at the husband's passing. After all, he had been through so much. How did you feel?" "It can sometimes be confusing that you feel comforted that your wife no longer has to suffer yet also feel that you would do anything to have her back." Grieving persons often have conflicting emotions and only after clarifying them, understanding them as part and parcel of grieving, and accepting them, can they move on with their lives.

Strategy 2f: Consider possible ways for the client to become involved with others. As the older client begins to come to terms with the death of the loved one and is less depressed, it is usually easier to think about ways to reestablish relationships or initiate new ones. One challenge for widowed older persons is that when their spouse was alive they frequently socialized with other older couples. A complaint that we frequently hear, especially from older women, is that they do not feel comfortable socializing with older couples. "I'm a third wheel." "A single woman is a threat to other women—she might steal a friend's husband." "My presence reminds them that they will become widowed too." Though these concerns sometimes reflect the client's own difficulty in coming to terms with a changed social status, we also believe that older people correctly perceive that some older couples prefer to primarily socialize with other couples and not single individuals. The therapist encourages the older client to take stock of existing relationships and new possibilities. Logical options include increased involvement in existing activities that offer opportunities for social interaction (e.g., attendance at religious services and associated social activities; greater involvement with children, grandchildren, siblings, or other relatives) and engagement in new activities (e.g., senior citizen center, volunteer opportunities, high school or university extension courses, group travel). The therapist needs to take into account the client's past history of social and interpersonal involvements rather than, for example, assume that all older adults would welcome spending time at a senior center. Some older adults may be interested in dating again and possible means of doing this might be explored. We find that there are an increasing number of formal and informal venues for meeting other older single adults, including those sponsored by churches or synagogues, YMCA/YMHA, commercial establishments, and the Internet. In larger cities there are some organizations for older gay and lesbian adults that offer opportunities for same-sex companionship.

CONTINUATION OF THE CASE OF GLORIA JOHNSON

The initial sessions of treatment of this case were discussed in chapter 5 (this volume). To recap: Mrs. Johnson was diagnosed with major depression, single episode, mild following the deaths of her brother and sister-in-law from AIDS. Marital tension with her husband increased while her relatives were dying and became more pronounced when she became seriously depressed following their deaths. The identified problem areas were grief and interpersonal role dispute.

Intermediate Sessions

Sessions 4, 5, 6. The therapist encouraged Mrs. Johnson to talk about her relationship with her brother and sister-in-law. She spoke lovingly of her brother whom she described as bright, sophisticated, and successful with a "great sense of humor." Their years growing up together were challenging as the family had little income. She told a memorable story of how her brother volunteered to use his paper-route money to pay for dance lessons she dearly wanted that her parents could not afford. "He was a gem." She liked her sister-in-law. During child rearing years, Mrs. Johnson and her family would often go on outings with her brother's family. In later years, Mrs. Johnson and her husband frequently socialized with her brother and sister-in-law. In subsequent sessions the therapist continued to inquire about depressive symptoms that did not appear to abate. Mrs. Johnson continued to be critical of herself for lack of initiative in doing household tasks and failure to respond to requests by friends to socialize. The therapist reminded her that she was still experiencing the effects of a depressive illness, that in due time it should improve, but that in the short run it was okay to do less. She reluctantly agreed to hire a cleaning woman "just for now."

The therapist found that Mrs. Johnson seemed most comfortable talking about her relationship with her brother and sister-in-law prior to their illnesses. As the therapist steered her to a discussion of the period of her relatives' failing health, she would move away from the topic. The therapist pointed this out. Mrs. Johnson acknowledged that she was doing this and how painful it was to discuss this topic. "I understand that this is hard for you but it is important for us to discuss this very difficult period. I will encourage you to do this. If the discussion becomes too painful let me know and we will slow things down." Though it is important for the therapist to respect the client's reluctance to proceed, it is also important for the therapist to communicate that the discussion must happen so the client can get at the source of the depression.

Session 7. Mrs. Johnson began the painful process of recounting the circumstances of her relatives' illnesses. "My sister-in-law just didn't look right. I keep telling her to go to the doctor. Finally she did and the doctor said that her lymph nodes were enlarged but the doctor couldn't figure out why. Then my brother began to complain he was feeling weak. At first I just thought he was trying to call attention to himself. He began to lose weight. He went to his cardiologist. He had had open heart surgery several years earlier and wondered whether he was having heart problems again. The doctor said his heart was fine." The therapist asked her what she was feeling at this time. "I thought they should go to the Mayo Clinic." "But how were you feeling?" asked the therapist. "I felt scared."

Session 8. The therapist completed the Hamilton Rating Scale for Depression (HRSD) on which Mrs. Johnson had a score of 20 which was higher than on initial evaluation. She attributed the increased score to a dispute with her husband in the past week. The therapist encouraged her to describe in detail the circumstances of the dispute. "I really felt we needed to go to a church social event because I was on the committee that organized it. He complained that he hated these events. I told him he was never there for me and began to list all of the disappointing things he had done. He said he wasn't going to listen to the same old complaints again, got in the car, and went somewhere. In the end, neither of us went to the event." The therapist pointed out that in view of the fact she continued to experience the effects of a depressive illness it must have been very difficult for Mrs. Johnson to mobilize herself to attend the event, and that her husband's reluctance to attend must have been disappointing and frustrating. Using IPT's communication analysis technique, the therapist helped Mrs. Johnson understand where "communication broke down," reviewed how she had successfully handled disputes with her husband in the past, and used role-playing to reenact the situation in a way that was less likely to lead to an increase in conflict. "I know that when I criticize him he just clams up. I guess it would have been better to say, 'I know you don't like these events and appreciate that you've gone in the past. Would you go with me tonight? We'll only stay an hour. Would you like to go out to dinner afterward?'" Mrs. Johnson acknowledged that since the onset of her depression she was more irritable and that it was harder for her to "take the high road" in disputes with her husband.

Sessions 9, 10, 11. Mrs. Johnson said she had apologized to her husband for being short-tempered with him. "He really appreciated that and we had a pretty good week." In this session, after reviewing the status of Mrs. Johnson's dispute with her husband, the therapist encouraged Mrs. Johnson to discuss in detail events surrounding her brother and sister-in-law's illnesses. She said it was painful to do this but would do her best. "And so someone said that they should go see an infectious disease specialist. They had been to South America on a trip and maybe they picked something up that was causing their health problems. When my sister-in-law called me with the news that they had AIDS, I was just floored. I was sure there was a mistake." The therapist inquired about the likely reason for the infection. "That was a mystery. My brother said that he must have contracted it during a blood transfusion during his heart surgery but the doctor said the blood had been screened for HIV. Until the very end my brother said that is how he contracted AIDS even though the doctor kept telling him that wasn't possible." Mrs. Johnson began the painful process of describing the physical decline of her brother and sister-in-law. The therapist encouraged her to speak about this and the feelings surrounding the events in detail. This discussion extended over several sessions and was obviously emotionally painful for Mrs. Johnson to recount.

She was frequently tearful as she recalled a succession of illnesses and health crises for her brother and sister-in-law. Because they became ill prior to the availability of protease inhibitors, few effective medications for AIDS were available. "My brother seemed to get sickest the fastest and was in and out of hospitals. He looked just awful and I'll bet he lost 40 pounds. It broke my heart to see him slipping away. At the end he was covered with those red cancerous spots. But even to the end my brother used his humor to deal with things. He joked about those spots but I could hardly look at him. I didn't even want to touch him. I feel ashamed about that. But that is the truth."

"And then the end came. At the funeral everyone asked what he died from and I lied. I said he had a rare blood disease. I hated myself for lying. I hated them for asking. I even hated God for doing this to us. My sister-in-law had to come to the funeral in a wheelchair. Can you imagine? Can you imagine?"

"But of course it wasn't over. My sister-in-law kept going downhill. In a few months she was dead. Another funeral. More lies. 'Isn't it just a terrible shame that you lost both of them in such a short period of time?' people would say. 'You don't know the half of it!' I wanted to shout. 'No, you don't know anything.'" The therapist asked how she was able to manage so much for so long. Mrs. Johnson said she just tried not to think about things and do what she needed to do to get through the day.

Session 12. Mrs. Johnson said that problems had flared up again with her husband. The therapist helped her to clarify the issue, her expectations of her husband, and her options to change things. She said a recurring issue was that she expected him to accompany her to events that he often didn't like. In recent weeks she had been feeling less depressed and was beginning to resume some of her social involvements. "I wanted to go to a play but he didn't. That led to a fight." Exploring this issue, Mrs. Johnson acknowledged her husband always hated plays but would go only if she badgered him. She acknowledged that an evening of forced socialization was unpleasant for both her and her husband. "But a husband should accompany his wife, yes?" Her expectations around this were explored and she began to entertain other options such as going to events alone or with a friend or other family member. She also identified things that her husband enjoyed doing with her, such as going out to dinner. She said that she would try to back off from putting pressure on her husband to attend events he didn't like and try to do more things that he enjoyed.

Session 13. Mrs. Johnson said that things were going more smoothly with her husband and that she felt less depressed and more hopeful. "But there's one more chapter of this AIDS drama I think I can tell you now. I told you that my brother said he contracted AIDS from a heart operation. I wanted to believe that and I kept telling myself that tests for HIV in blood couldn't be 100% accurate. In the back of my mind I wondered if that was the case. After my sister-in-law died, her daughter and I started the process of disposing of their things before we sold the house. As I was going through my brother's clothes I found several matchbooks that had sexual pictures printed on them and what seemed to be a name of a club. I showed them to my niece who grew very silent. We finished things up and a few days later she called me and told me the matchbooks were from a private club that was known to cater to sexual encounters between its members. My niece was so upset and angry about this. We never talked about it again."

The therapist asked Mrs. Johnson how she felt about this. "I was so angry at my brother. To think that he had sexual relations with other women, got AIDS, and then infected his wife. I hated my brother. I hated my brother so much. I told my husband but I don't think he wanted to deal with it. I hated my brother and missed him at the same time. I was glad he had died because he had done this and yet wished so much he was still here. I was so confused. I just stopped thinking about it and then I got depressed." The relief Mrs. Johnson felt in telling this "final chapter of the AIDS drama" was palpable. "You're feeling less depressed now," commented the therapist, "as you've honestly reckoned with the painful realities you've faced and the complex emotions you've felt."

Termination

Session 14. Mrs. Johnson spoke more of her feelings about her brother. She said she always wondered if he had been faithful to his wife—"you know how men are." "How do you feel now after telling me about how he likely contracted HIV?" asked the therapist. "Relief, sadness. I love my brother. He made a wrong decision. I just wish he had been more careful." The therapist reminded Mrs. Johnson of the two remaining sessions and asked how she felt about ending. She said that it was hard because there had been so many endings. The therapist counseled her that ending psychotherapy can be a time for another sort of grieving and that it was normal to have feelings about that ending. "You and I have been through so much together," remarked Mrs. Johnson.

Sessions 15, 16. Mrs. Johnson said that things were going more smoothly between her and her husband. "He says that I seem more relaxed." Mrs. Johnson said she felt nervous about ending therapy and wondered how she could be able to handle things on her own. The therapist again reminded her that this was normal. At the beginning of the 16th session the therapist readministered the HRSD, on which the client had a score of 6. "As you recall, when you started therapy your score was 18 and now it is 6, which means you are in the nondepressed range. Also, your symptoms have improved and you no longer have a major depression." Mrs. Johnson acknowledged that she felt much better and seemed relieved to know that she no longer had a major depression.

The therapist then reviewed the course of psychotherapy, emphasizing the active efforts that she had made to deal with depression and the problems that accompanied it. "Your depressive illness followed a remarkably difficult life situation that involved the loss of two people very important to you from a societally stigmatizing illness that is associated with a myriad of health consequences. Psychologically, grief became more complicated because it appears that your brother engaged in sexual behavior outside of the marriage from which he contracted AIDS. As if things weren't difficult enough, your depressive illness put a strain on your marriage at a time when you most needed your husband. You have made many efforts to untangle the painful stories that you called the 'AIDS drama.' It was only by recalling and emotionally processing this trauma that you were able to move on with your life. At the same time you reviewed problems in your marital life, examined expectations, communicated with your husband, and went on to make some changes that made a difference. You're returning to social involvements that you had previously enjoyed. You've been courageous in your efforts and I want to convey my deep respect for what you've done."

Case Commentary

The case of Mrs. Johnson is a dramatic story of complicated grief. Rarely do we see cases in our outpatient geriatric clinic in which AIDS has so powerfully affected the lives of older adults. The dynamics of Mrs. Johnson's complicated grief, however, are familiar to Clougherty, who worked on a research study of IPT for the treatment of depression in young adults with AIDS (Markowitz et al., 1999). Parents of study patients often had to deal with the emotional consequences of illness, loss of an adult child, and the social shame and isolation of not being able to be candid with others about AIDS. IPT treatment in this case focused on facilitation of the mourning process and reestablishment of interests and relationships for what was lost. Grief was facilitated by the therapist's sharp focus on details of the physical deterioration and death of her brother and sister-in-law. Within the context of a nonjudgmental therapeutic relationship Mrs. Johnson could increasingly be candid about what she had gone through, and eventually share the most painful secret of the AIDS drama: that her brother appeared to have contracted AIDS through sexual relations outside of his marriage. Although a relationship with her brother and sister-in-law could never be truly substituted, resolution of depression facilitated reengagement in social activities that had previously been important to her. Within the secondary problem area, interpersonal role disputes, Mrs. Johnson was able to identify certain expectations about her husband related to social involvements, modify those expectations and some patterns of communication, and therefore improve marital relations.

CASE EXAMPLE: PETER O'BRIEN

Mr. O'Brien was a 75-year-old, Catholic, Caucasian man who had been widowed about 6 months. The onset of a major depressive disorder, moderate, recurrent had occurred about 2 months prior to evaluation. The depression followed a dispute with his deceased wife's children over his wife's estate. Medical problems included enlarged prostate, high cholesterol, and borderline hypertension. Among prescribed medications, he was taking a benzodiazepine for anxiety. An antidepressant medication was recommended but he declined. Mr. O'Brien agreed to consider antidepressant medication if his depression did not improve. The interpersonal inventory revealed that he had a good relationship with his deceased wife who died after a 3-year struggle with breast cancer. His first wife had died from liver cancer 30 years ago. He had one surviving sister with whom he had minimal contact and an adult daughter who lived on the West Coast. He was in regular contact by telephone with his daughter with whom he described having a close relationship. His recently deceased wife had three children by another marriage, with whom he had had "cordial" relations until her death. After her death, relations seriously deteriorated. He said that he was friendly with a female neighbor who had been supportive to him during his wife's illness. On the whole, the interpersonal inventory revealed a man who had primarily organized his emotional life around his wife and daughter and who had no substantive connections with friends or other family. The HRSD score obtained during the first session was 23, which indicated *significant depression*. Identified problem areas included grief and interpersonal role dispute.

Intermediate Sessions

Session 4. The therapist reviewed Mr. O'Brien's depressive symptoms. Symptoms appeared to have worsened in the prior week because he had received a letter from a lawyer representing his deceased wife's children. The letter directed Mr. O'Brien to vacate a beach house that had been owned by his wife because it was claimed that the house now belonged to her children. "That's my house too. It's true my wife bought it before we were married but I totally remodeled it over the years." Mr. O'Brien was angry and upset by the letter. "She was barely in the ground when they told me that the beach house was theirs. I could hardly believe it. First I told them that this wasn't the time to talk about it. But they kept hammering me. I finally told them to go to hell." He was so puzzled why they were so insistent on claiming the beach house. It appeared to the therapist that grieving his wife's death became complicated once the dispute emerged. Dealing with the dispute seemed to be the first order of business in the therapy and was the focus of several of the initial intermediate sessions.

From an IPT perspective, the stage of the dispute with his wife's children was that of renegotiation with use of the therapeutic strategy to calm down participants to facilitate resolution. Although the primary issue in the dispute appeared to be ownership of the beach house, the therapist explored whether other issues existed. Had the children laid claim to other assets? Had there been past disputes with the children about money? Were there past interpersonal issues with the children for which the beach house dispute might be a proxy? Mr. O'Brien said that after their mother's death he gladly gave her children personal items of their mother that they requested. He indicated that they had not requested other assets and could not recall past problems with the children over money. The therapist asked if he had spoken with the children recently. Mr. O'Brien said they would not take his calls since he told one of the children to "go to hell." Options (i.e., continued silence, direct communication with the children, and contact with them through a lawyer) were reviewed with the therapist and Mr. O'Brien decided that he should retain the services of a lawyer.

Session 5. Mr. O'Brien reported that he met with a lawyer who reviewed the letter he had received from his wife's children's lawyer. His own lawyer felt that because he was the surviving spouse, the beach house was indeed owned by Mr. O'Brien despite the claim of his wife's children. The therapist encouraged Mr. O'Brien to review his options at this point. He decided that he would call one of his wife's children to arrange an informal meeting to discuss the situation.

Session 6. Mr. O'Brien said that he had spoken to one of the children who said that their mother had promised the house to them. He visibly appeared more depressed and said he felt more discouraged and hopeless. Mr. O'Brien expressed surprise because his wife had never told him she had promised the beach house to the children. The therapist inquired about what legal planning his wife had made prior to her death. "None. She wouldn't talk about it. I really didn't know how to bring the topic up but when I did, she wouldn't discuss things. I tried several times. She said that there was no need to discuss this topic because she would be getting better." The therapist inquired whether she may have had conversations with her children about the beach house prior to her death. He said he didn't know. The therapist encouraged Mr. O'Brien to review options to deal with the dispute. Mr. O'Brien decided to call a meeting with his lawyer, his wife's children's lawyer, and his wife's children.

Session 7. Although the children were reluctant to do so, a meeting was arranged. The children said that the beach house was very important to them. They had wonderful memories of summers at the beach house and it was a connection not only to their mother but also to their deceased father who had originally built the house. They said that when their mother was dying she told them that the house was theirs after her death. In fact, they said, she had repeated this several times. Both lawyers agreed that legally the house belonged to Mr. O'Brien, a fact that the children reluctantly accepted. At the end of the meeting the children were obviously disappointed but treated Mr. O'Brien respectfully. Later in the session, Mr. O'Brien began to talk about the frustration he felt over his wife's unwillingness not only to make advance plans for her death but to acknowledge how sick she was. "After she finished chemotherapy for the second time, the doctors told us that the cancer wasn't going into remission and that it didn't make sense to pursue further treatment. I knew what that meant. But she kept telling me that everything would get better." The therapist asked what she told friends and family about the condition. "Oh, she told everyone including her children that she was getting better and that the treatment was working. But that just wasn't true." The therapist asked how he felt about this. "Frustrated." "Were you annoyed or even angry at her about this?" inquired the therapist. "How could I be angry at someone who was dying?" The therapist provided some education about the complexity of feelings that often accompany care for a person who is very ill. In IPT it is important that the therapist not shy away from exploring feelings of anger that the client may feel toward the deceased. Discussion of angry feelings is initially difficult for the client but may be necessary for resolution of grief.

Session 8. Mr. O'Brien's depressive symptoms were significantly reduced. On the HRSD he had a score of 11, which indicated *mild depression*. He acknowledged feeling better and relieved that the legal dispute with his wife's children seemed to be at an end. Yet he felt bad for the children too. Doubts lingered about whether indeed his wife had told the children that they would get the beach house on her death. Why would she talk openly about death with her children when she told him that she was getting better? Was she saying one thing to them and another thing to him? At this point he shared his feelings of anger. "Why did she leave me in this position? I asked her to make plans but she wouldn't." He said that his wife had forbade him to tell anyone that she was as sick as she really was. "She even said I couldn't tell my daughter she had cancer." In desperation one day, he blurted out the truth to a neighbor who was a nurse. "It all came out. I told her everything. She listened very patiently and helped me to think about how I could better deal with the situation. When I told my wife I had talked with the neighbor she was very angry at me and said that I betrayed her. I felt guilty but I kept talking to the neighbor. I needed to talk to someone."

Session 9. The therapist encouraged Mr. O'Brien to talk about his relationship with his wife. They had had a good marriage and he looked to her for emotional support. In fact, he had met his wife at a bereavement group shortly after both of their spouses died when they were younger. He described himself as being "in shock" when he learned that he would again have to care for a wife with cancer. "Lightning isn't supposed to strike twice, eh?" His first wife died quickly after diagnosis. He was able to distract himself with work and was comforted in finding a new partner so shortly after his first wife died. The therapist also encouraged Mr. O'Brien to talk about what it was like caring for his wife when she was ill. "At first, it wasn't so bad and we were hopeful she would beat the cancer. Toward the end it got harder and harder." "What were the hardest parts of caring for your wife?" asked the therapist. He vaguely referred to "dealing with doctors," "paying medical bills," and doing "all the housework."

Sessions 10, 11. In the next sessions the therapist pulled for details of what it was like to care for his wife in her final days. Was she at home? Could she get out of bed? What did she look like? Slowly Mr. O'Brien described how his wife spent her final days at home. She had lost an enormous amount of weight, was incontinent, and was, at times, delirious. He recalled "the smell of death" in the room and his reluctance to change his wife's adult diapers. He described these events with considerable emotion as he visibly tried to hold back tears. "And where did she die?" asked the therapist. "She died at home. She seemed to have trouble breathing and I called the doctor. I held her hand, telling her that everything would be all right. She opened her eyes and looked at me and then she stopped breathing. Suddenly it was quiet and I realized she was gone. I just sat by her bed and waited for the doctor."

Session 12. Mr. O'Brien appeared even less depressed than he was at Week 8. He began to discuss plans to visit his daughter on the West Coast and spoke of the possibility of moving there. He said that he had thought about the conflict over the beach house and that he was willing to sell the house to his wife's adult children for "a very fair price" if they want to buy it. He was reminded that four therapy sessions remained.

Before the next scheduled session he called and said that he had spoken with his daughter and decided to make a trip to the West Coast to visit her. His daughter said that this was a good time to visit and he had arranged an inexpensive plane fare. A psychotherapy appointment was set up on his return.

Session 13. On his return, Mr. O'Brien reported that he had a very enjoyable visit with his daughter and her family. They talked about his wife's illness and death, and his daughter had an opportunity to talk about what it was like to lose her mother. They also discussed the conflict with his wife's children regarding the beach house. "I realized my wife wanted to please all of us and probably told her kids they could have the beach house because she knew how much it meant to them. She left me with a mess, however, because she wouldn't work out all of this with us together. Maybe she was even trying to protect me from the idea that she was dying. I admit that I felt angry about that even if she was sick." He and his daughter talked further about what would be a fair price for the beach house and made an initial call to his wife's children. They were receptive to his call and said they would think about it.

Termination

Session 14. In the session the therapist raised the issue that there were two more remaining sessions. Mr. O'Brien said that he wanted to take a trip to Florida the following week and therefore would not be able to take part in two more sessions. They renegotiated the following week's appointment so that they could meet prior to his departure. The therapist asked about Mr. O'Brien's feelings about ending therapy. He said that it had been helpful to him and that he felt confident that he would be fine. He felt better, the dispute with his wife's children seemed headed for an amicable ending, and he had had an opportunity to talk with the therapist as well as his daughter about the stress of caring for his wife.

Session 15. In the final session, Mr. O'Brien scored 4 on the HRSD, which was in the nondepressed range for the scale. "Your score has gone from 23 to 4 and you no longer have symptoms of a major depression. You've worked very hard in therapy to deal with the dispute with your wife's children regarding the beach house and talked about the stress and pain of caring for your wife. Dealing with your wife's death was made more complicated because of the dispute with her children but also because your wife didn't do the best job in planning for her death. She was secretive about how ill she was. This put you in a difficult position because she didn't even want you talking to anyone about her health problems. This secretiveness seeded later problems—problems that you have actively dealt with." Mr. O'Brien said that he was a "little nervous" about ending and asked if on his return he could meet with the therapist one more time if he needed to. The therapist assured him that he could. Mr. O'Brien never set up another appointment.

Case Commentary

The mourning process was stalled and complicated for Mr. O'Brien because of the dispute with his deceased wife's children over property. The dispute itself, however, appeared to emerge from his wife's unwillingness or inability to makes plans for her death, thus leaving Mr. O'Brien with what he called a "mess." Success in his efforts to resolve the dispute with his wife's children took emotional pressure off Mr. O'Brien, with subsequent improvement in his depressive symptoms. The discussion with his deceased wife's children, however, raised questions about what she had told them before she died and brought into sharper focus her failure to plan for her death.

The therapist facilitated the mourning process by helping Mr. O'Brien discuss his relationship with his wife but, most important, what it was like caring for his wife while she was dying. IPT's techniques of exploration, encouragement of affect, and clarification were integral to this process. Negative as well as positive feelings toward his wife were evident during this discussion. As Mr. O'Brien came to terms with his wife's death and was less depressed, he began to consider options for the reestablishment of a new life without his wife.

CONCLUDING COMMENTARY

In clinical practice, we find that interpersonal role disputes are often part of complicated grief. Unresolved interpersonal and family issues can come to the fore at a painful and poignant time for survivors of the deceased. Following the death of a loved one, emotions are raw. Some individuals make hurtful remarks toward others that would not have been made under other circumstances, or remarks from others are interpreted in negative ways that had not been intended. The deceased's property can become a proxy for long-standing, unresolved issues between parties. As illustrated in Mr. O'Brien's case, the deceased's behavior during the dying process may lay the groundwork for conflict after death. As in Mrs. Johnson's case, relations may be strained between the grieving individual who is now depressed and significant others. Others may view a prolonged process of grief as self-indulgent and evidence of emotional weakness. Psychotherapy is a place where a frank discussion of issues can take place. Although some individuals may want to shy away from the painful feelings associated with complicated bereavement, the therapist gently but firmly guides the client through a process that can be emotionally healing and result in improvement of depressive symptoms and establishment of a meaningful life without the deceased.

7

INTERPERSONAL ROLE DISPUTES

As noted in chapter 1 (this volume), most older people experience reasonably satisfying family and social relationships. This fact stands in contrast to the stereotypical characterizations sometimes made of older people as socially isolated, lonely, and abandoned by their children (Shanas, 1979). Yet some older adults have chronic interpersonal problems. Those with chronic interpersonal problems tend to have personality disorders (Rosowsky, Abrams, & Zweig, 1999). Most older adults have occasional difficulties with family members and friends and are able to deal with them in a manner that preserves the relationship. Though disputes with significant others can be experienced as stressful and may be accompanied by some anxiety or depressive symptoms, they do not typically lead to major depression or adjustment disorder. For others, however, the emergence or exacerbation of an interpersonal dispute does lead to a clinically significant depression (Hinrichsen & Emery, 2005). See chapters 2 and 3 (this volume) for a discussion of the interpersonal antecedents of depression.

In our clinical practice with older adults, interpersonal role disputes typically involve spouse or partner, adult child, or sibling. Sometimes disputes are with a friend or parent of advanced years. Among long-married persons, chronic marital problems can become exacerbated by late-life stressors. For married persons with historically good marital relationships, a dispute may be triggered by retirement, new or additional responsibilities for care of the spouse, problems in the lives of adult children or grandchildren, or other problems. For some, the chief interpersonal problem is contending with the difficulties associated with the spouse's major depression. As noted earlier, research has found that compared with younger couples, older dyads generally manage marital difficulties in ways that reduce the likelihood of conflict and, when conflict does arise, they more readily deescalate the conflict to establish harmony (Carstensen, Gottman, & Levenson, 1995). Some older adults are not married but have long-standing relationships. Over the years, we have noted an increase in the number of older clients in nonmarital dyads and anticipate that entry of baby boomers in geriatric practice in a few years will make these even more common. Nonmarried dyadic relationships take a variety of forms including heterosexual couples who chose not to marry or partnered gay and lesbian older persons (Kimmel, 2002). We also find some older adults who have had long-standing relationships with married persons. Others have newly established relationships, and clinically relevant problems reflect those that are often experienced by newly coupled individuals. We occasionally see married older adults with spouses with severe dementia in nursing homes who have started romantic relationships with other persons and who struggle with issues over their need for intimacy versus guilt in establishing a relationship prior to the spouse's death.

For older adults who have disputes with adult children, problems sometimes arise in the context of relationships that historically have been troubled. Typical issues involve differences over frequency of contact or visiting, the adult child's style of raising grandchildren, and the extent of help provided to the aging parent who is caring for an infirm spouse. Interpersonal tensions may be exacerbated by the emergence of psychiatric illness in the older adult. Some older adults have children with psychiatric difficulties, substance abuse problems, medical problems, histories of erratic employment, chronic financial difficulties, and current or past problems with the legal system. Sometimes adult children with problems live with the older adult, a situation that can increase stress. In fact, in our outpatient geriatric psychiatry clinic we have a psychotherapy group just for older adults with children who have psychiatric or other life problems.

GOALS AND STRATEGIES IN IPT TREATMENT OF INTERPERSONAL ROLE DISPUTES

As noted in the outline (see Exhibit 7.1), the goals of interpersonal psychotherapy (IPT) in this problem area involve identification of the dispute, clarification of the stage of the dispute, choice of a plan or plans of action to deal with it, and modification of expectations about the relationship or a change in problematic communication behavior in an attempt to

EXHIBIT 7.1

Outline of Interpersonal Psychotherapy for Major Depression

B. Interpersonal Role Disputes
  1. Goals
      a. Identify dispute.
      b. Choose plan of action.
      c. Modify expectations or faulty communication to bring about a satisfactory resolution.
  2. Strategies
      a. Review depressive symptoms.
      b. Relate symptom onset to overt or covert dispute with significant other with whom patient is currently involved.
      c. Determine stage of dispute:
          i. renegotiation (calm down participants to facilitate resolution);
          ii. impasse (increase disharmony in order to reopen negotiation);
          iii. dissolution (assist mourning).
      d. Understand how nonreciprocal role expectations relate to dispute:
          i. What are the issues in the dispute?
          ii. What are differences in expectations and values?
          iii. What are the options?
          iv. What is the likelihood of finding alternatives?
          v. What resources are available to bring about change in the relationship?
      e. Are there parallels in other relationships?
          i. What is the patient gaining?
          ii. What unspoken assumptions lie behind the patient's behavior?
      f. How is the dispute perpetuated?

Note. From *Comprehensive Guide to Interpersonal Psychotherapy* (p. 23), by M. M. Weissman, J. C. Markowitz, and G. L. Klerman, 2000, New York: Basic Books. Copyright 2000 by Basic Books. Reprinted with permission.

bring about resolution. For example, in the case of a marital dispute, at the end of the initial sessions sometimes we more broadly refer to these goals by indicating that "one of the major goals of the therapy will be that you have a better handle on your difficulties with your wife." By characterizing the general thrust of work within this problem domain, we leave room for a variety of outcomes including reestablishment of productive communication and cooperation between the parties, a change in expectations about the relationship that reduces the client's persistent and ultimately frustrating efforts to "change the other person" or some aspect of the relationship that is unlikely to change, or end of the relationship. The emphasis of IPT in this problem area is on what the client can actively do to maximize the likelihood that relationship issues can be resolved. If issues cannot be changed, the client then is encouraged to actively change his or her own expectations. As can be seen, the emphasis is on the client as an active player in dealing with a problematic relationship. This stance is in contrast to the passive sense of defeat that many depressed clients have when an important relationship has not gone well. We have found that even for those for whom the troubled relationship did not improve after their best efforts, the act of trying is therapeutic. Although some individuals with a dispute assert at the beginning of therapy that the other party is solely to blame, they privately wonder whether they could have managed interpersonal difficulties with more wisdom, care, and patience. Clients who use the IPT strategies for this problem area are more likely to approach the relationship problem in a manner that involves "taking the high ground," "giving it my best shot," or "trying my best."

Strategy 2a: Review depressive symptoms and **Strategy 2b:** Relate symptom onset to overt or covert dispute with significant other with whom patient is currently involved. Depressive symptoms and their relationship with the dispute are ascertained in the initial sessions. The association between onset of depression and the dispute bears frequent repeating during the middle sessions. Increases or decreases in depressive symptoms that follow recent relationship problems or improvement in problems are explicitly pointed out. The message to the client is that "your experiences with people affect the way you feel."

Strategy 2c: Determine stage of dispute. A determination of the stage of the dispute guides therapeutic efforts. In the renegotiation stage of a dispute, frequent arguments are evidence of active discord between the parties. In this stage, arguments may emerge around the central issues or issues that are in dispute or around other topics that may be a proxy for the larger issues. Both parties may be especially sensitive to comments and behaviors from the other that can be a trigger for arguments. A mental recounting of recent incidents and a cataloguing of the other party's faults are associated with feelings of anger. The prime strategy at this stage of the dispute is to encourage the client to calm angry feelings and behave in a manner that makes it less likely that his or her own behavior will trigger angry feelings in the other party. At the impasse stage of the dispute, one or both parties have stopped trying to address or even communicate about issues of concern. Klerman and Weissman speak of the "cold marriage" as an example of this (Klerman, Weissman, Rounsaville, & Chevron, 1984). For this current generation of older adults in which divorce is less common than in subsequent generations, long-standing, unhappy marriages are seen in clinical practice. Some older people characterize their relationship with the spouse as having been unsatisfactory for much of the marriage. Divorce was not seriously considered for religious, social, or economic reasons. For older adults, the economic consequences of divorce can be devastating to both parties, leaving even middle-class individuals in precarious financial circumstances. Some older couples agree to remain together for economic reasons while acknowledging that they are mismatched.

Similarly long-standing disputes may exist between older people and their adult children. Several of our clients have had only sporadic contact with an adult child. A series of disputes earlier in life were followed by disengagement on the part of one or both parties. One client described a 25-year estrangement from her daughter as "an open wound" and continued to hope that at the end of her life the relationship would be healed despite evidence to the contrary. The prime strategy for individuals in the impasse stage is to facilitate communication about the issue of dispute. Opening up discussion will almost inevitably increase expression of anger and disappointment on the part of both parties. Although in this circumstance angry affect needs to be carefully managed so that it is less likely to lead to an even greater impasse, disharmony may get a dialogue going that might lead to another effort to deal with issues of common concern.

With some older couples we find that disputes may emerge against the backdrop of a marriage that has been at an impasse for many years. Discouraged that years of efforts to deal with relationship problems have not worked, each member of the older couple finds separate social and recreational outlets. Conflict is minimized by minimal contact. However, retirement or the onset of health problems in one or both older adults may lead to conflict that has been avoided for many years. For example, one older couple seen in clinical practice had many years of an impasse that erupted into conflict when the husband began to have increasing medical problems. His need for care brought them into sustained contact with each other. His wife resented the care she was required to provide to him and during one dispute he threw her to the ground and began choking her. They came for treatment with hopes of returning to their status quo relationship impasse. The conflict, however, provided a vehicle for discussing some long-standing problems and better accommodation to each other that resulted in better though far-from-ideal relations.

Occasionally, a client believes that a problematic relationship must end and the client is seeking help in psychotherapy with terminating the relationship. At first, the IPT therapist must be vigilant about the possibility that the client's conviction that there is no hope for improvement in the relationship primarily reflects feelings of hopelessness and helplessness that are common in depression. It is important that the therapist carefully explore the history of the relationship that the client might not have considered. Some clients begin therapy with the hope that relationship problems can be successfully addressed but then come to the conclusion that relationship dissolution is the only viable option. In the end, it is the client's decision about how to proceed with the problematic relationship. We have found that even in cases where the client decides to end the relationship, the process of coming to this conclusion can be empowering.

Strategy 2d: Understand how nonreciprocal role expectations relate to dispute. This strategy is at the heart of the IPT treatment of interpersonal role disputes. What are the issues in the dispute? Sometimes the answer to this question is fairly clear from the beginning of therapy. At other times clarification requires considerable discussion within therapy. The issue or issues in the relationship become conflated with negative portrayals of the character or intentions of the significant other. Or, some clients find it hard to move beyond a telling of one episode after another in which they felt hurt by the other. At some point older clients are swimming in a sea of negative affect surrounded by the flotsam and jetsam of one unresolved problem after another. Older people in relationship impasse may find it hard to articulate the specific problems that led to the impasse—to extend the prior metaphor, they are frozen in a sea of disappointed expectations. Some clients may present a litany of problems and the therapist should identify the most important ones. As issues tied to the dispute become clearer, the therapy can shift to an understanding of differences in expectations and values. *Expectations* and *values* are neutral terms and can move the therapeutic discussion beyond blaming to a recognition that there are two parties to the dispute who bring different attitudes, life experiences, and interpersonal strengths and weaknesses. Often clients have not articulated expectations and values for themselves that are implicit in remarks they make. A comment such as "What kind of daughter does something like that?" could be followed by the therapist commenting, "What do you think your daughter should do?" Some clients have expectations that they never directly articulated to the other party. "Anybody should know that." The therapist might then explain that not everyone automatically understands what the other person wants. The therapist also facilitates the client's understanding of values and expectations of the other person. Clarification of values and expectations may be difficult because there will be a tendency to characterize the other person's expectations in a judgmental fashion. "Expectations? He expects me to pick up after him all the time. He's a slob." The therapist might ask the client what the other person might say about himself in an effort to clarify the other party's expectations and values. A shift in expectations and values at some point in the marriage may have occurred yet neither party discussed it. "I always did the shopping and cooking and cleaning. He's not working now. Why can't he help?"

After clarification of the issues, expectations, and values that are critical to the dispute, an exploration of options is initiated by the therapist. We believe this is the heart of IPT treatment for disputes. Exploration of options is an empowering strategy in which the client reviews what might be done to address the dispute. For those who choose to make efforts to engage in a dialogue with the other party, the IPT technique of communication analysis is especially helpful. Basic communication strategies such as finding the right time and place to have a conversation about problems (vs. raising them in the context of an angry argument), using *I* statements (vs. critical statements about what the other person has done), monitoring and managing angry emotions in the context of a discussion, and planning constructive and emotionally deescalating responses to provocative issues raised by the other party (vs. just seeing what happens) can powerfully facilitate a dialogue with the other party. Sometimes therapists forget that basic principles of communication are not known to all people, especially to those who have problem relationships. This generation of older adults grew up in a different, less psychologically minded culture compared with baby boomers and the generations that followed. Self-help books and talk shows on relationships were not part of their formative life experiences. Sometimes what appear to be fairly obvious ways to productively talk about interpersonal problems may not be so obvious to some older adults.

A companion technique is role-playing. We find that initially many older adults find role-playing awkward but with persistence most can be engaged in it. Older clients may feel embarrassed to role-play or disconcerted by how revealing of themselves the technique is. Role-playing may involve reenacting a recent argument or practicing a conversation with the other party about an issue of concern. Role-playing can better reveal the older client's communication deficits and skills as well as associated affect of which he or she may not be aware. A related technique is for the therapist to encourage the client to offer detailed descriptions of the back-and-forth of a recent disagreement. Some clients provide a global and often value-laden account of a recent difficulty. "It was the same old thing. He started criticizing me and I just walked out of the room." We push for details such as "What did he say exactly? What were his words?", "What did you say then?", and "What was the tone of your voice?"

Another option is for the other party to join in one or two IPT sessions. Meeting the other person may be very helpful to the therapist in understanding the other party's perspective and how the dyad communicates. As noted in chapter 3 (this volume), there is a conjoint form of IPT for interpersonal role disputes (Foley et al., 1989). In subsequent individual sessions the therapist can use observations from the conjoint meeting to help the client better deal with issues in the dispute. In general, relevant other or others may be invited to join in an IPT session.

What is the likelihood of finding alternatives? What resources are available to bring about change in the relationship? These IPT interpersonal role dispute strategies involve an honest reckoning of what the client feels capable of doing and what the other party is likely capable of doing. Though IPT aims at optimizing individuals' resources to successfully contend with role disputes, interpersonal capabilities and the ability to acquire interpersonal skills vary among people. The party to the dispute also may have limitations that make it unlikely that a productive conversation about common problems will occur. Some relationships may be beyond repair and dissolution may seem to be the best option. Although the therapist may hope to facilitate resolution of the dispute, ultimately resolution is the client's decision. On the other hand, the therapist must be vigilant about whether the client's pessimism about resolution represents a realistic appraisal of the situation or whether it reflects negativity that is often interwoven with depression.

Strategy 2e: Are there parallels in other relationships? In the initial sessions the interpersonal inventory will give valuable clues to characteristic patterns of relating to others. The client may or may not evidence problems in other relationships that parallel those with the party to the dispute. If parallels exist, the therapist points them out. Once a therapeutic relationship is established, most older clients are capable of hearing of the parallels from the therapist without perceiving the observation as criticism. Some clients are often critical of others, which seeds interpersonal friction. Although the focus of IPT is on the present, these expectations may have historical antecedents that are worth exploring as they are relevant to the identified problem(s). For example, an older IPT client had a dispute with her adult daughter over the frequency with which she visited the client's husband in the nursing home. She was also angry at nursing home staff for their failure to spend more time with her husband, her son for his infrequent invitations to his home, and her grandchildren for their failure to remember her birthday, and she had other related disappointments. Having learned in conducting the interpersonal inventory that the client had lost both of her parents in childhood and was raised reluctantly by an older sister, the therapist pursued a discussion of the possible significance of these early events to her in late life. The client said that she learned early in life that the only way to get what she needed was to "fight for it." She assumed that others would not be there for her and the only way to get what she needed was to demand it. Her demanding behavior paradoxically made it less likely that important people would be there for her. Alternative ways of getting what she wanted were pursued in therapy.

Strategy 2f: How is the dispute perpetuated? Focus on this question blends many of the above strategies in a way that the client can more fully reckon with expectations and values that drive and perpetuate interpersonal problems (and the assumptions that underlie them) as well as associated problematic communication behavior. With this understanding, the therapist encourages the client to make changes in expectations and behavior that promote a more successful resolution of the dispute. To ascertain how a dispute is perpetuated, the therapist must get detailed accounts of the client's weekly interactions with the other person in the dispute. Over time, a pattern may emerge that demonstrates the ways in which the dispute is perpetuated. Often, the client is unaware of this pattern and is surprised when the pattern is pointed out by the therapist. With this knowledge, however, the client may be able to attempt change in the relationship.

CONTINUATION OF THE CASE OF MARY RYAN

Discussion of the initial sessions of this case can be found in chapter 5 (this volume). To recap: Mrs. Ryan is a 79-year-old widowed woman who experienced the onset of a major depression following a dispute with her sister during a vacation to Ireland. She had a Hamilton Rating Scale for

Depression (HRSD) score of 22 (*significant depression*) at the beginning of psychotherapy. Her sister sprained her ankle during the vacation and insisted Mrs. Ryan accompany her home. Mrs. Ryan refused. On their return home her sister's displeasure with her was evident in her sister's refusal to speak with her at a family gathering and minimal communication with her at common church social events. She felt her efforts to mend the relationship were rebuffed by her sister.

Intermediate Sessions

Session 4. The therapist initially inquired about Mrs. Ryan's symptoms. She said she felt a little less anxious but continued to experience most of the depression-related symptoms she had reported in the first sessions. Mrs. Ryan complained that in the prior week she and her sister sat at the same table at a church social event and that her sister not only refused to speak with her but would not even make eye contact. She complained bitterly about her sister's behavior. "How could a sister do that?" "What kind of person is she?" "How dare she treat me that way!" Mrs. Ryan tried to draw the therapist into an acknowledgment that her sister was clearly wrong. The therapist tried to move the discussion to a better understanding of the issues in the dispute and differences in expectations and values that each party held. Mrs. Ryan, like many clients, initially found it difficult to look at the dispute from the other party's perspective and preferred to complain about her sister. The therapist inquired about what efforts she had made to resolve the dispute. She said several months earlier she had spoken with her sister at a family gathering in an effort to "make up." Despite her propensity to speak globally and vaguely about this encounter ("she was just impossible") the therapist gently pressed her for details of the conversation. It became evident that Mrs. Ryan had approached her sister defensively and critically. "I said to my sister, 'What's wrong with you? Why are you acting this way?' Her sister responded, 'What's wrong with me? What's wrong with you? You're selfish and don't care about anyone but yourself.'" The therapist asked whether she might have considered approaching her sister differently so that it was less likely the discussion would erupt into the dispute. Mrs. Ryan looked annoyed and commented to the therapist, "Whose side are you on anyway?" She felt that the therapist's inquiry connoted criticism of her. "Mrs. Ryan, I'm on your side. The reason I'm asking you these questions is to get a better sense of how you and your sister communicate. That's the only way I can understand where you and your sister get stuck in talking to each other. I'm on your side because I want to work with you to decrease your depression and improve the chances that you and your sister can resolve this difficulty. It's only in understanding the details of what happened that we can work together to change things." She seemed unconvinced.

Session 5. The therapist returned to Mrs. Ryan's concerns that the therapist was "siding" with her sister. Mrs. Ryan said that she had thought about what the therapist said and acknowledged that she might have handled things differently. "But you can see how stubborn my sister is, can't you?" The therapist said that clearly there were very strong feelings on both sides and that these feelings made it all the more difficult for either of them to calmly talk about the problems in their relationship. As is the case with many clients, Mrs. Ryan wanted the therapist to side with her, yet to have done so would have meant that Mrs. Ryan could not have understood her sister's position. The past relationship between Mrs. Ryan and her sister was explored. She said that her sister had always been the dominant person in their relationship ever since childhood. She described her sister as "self-confident" and "in charge" whereas she portrayed herself as "lacking in self-confidence" and "unsure of myself." Throughout much of their adult lives she felt comfortable being the little sister to the older sister although she acknowledged that, at times, she was angry at her sister's behavior. "But I kept my mouth shut. I wanted peace." The relationship with her sister began to slowly change after the death of Mrs. Ryan's husband. "As I told you, it was very hard to get over my husband's death." She described her relationship with her husband in ways that paralleled her relationship with her sister. She generally went along with what her husband wanted, depended on him to make the major decisions in their lives, and was reluctant to "speak my mind." The therapist noted this relationship pattern to the patient and she acknowledged that throughout much of her life she had played "second fiddle" to other people. She said that after her husband's death she turned to her sister and brother-in-law for guidance and help but that at some point she was forced to handle many things herself. "I was surprised I did all the things that needed to be done like paying the bills, handling money, calling the plumber." Her self-confidence began to build and she began to think of herself differently. She also began to notice some tension in her relationship with her sister. "I didn't want to be the little sister anymore. I sometimes answered back to my sister and she didn't like that."

Sessions 6 and 7. In the next two sessions the therapist encouraged further discussion of her relationship with her sister and how their role relationship with each other had slowly changed over the years. Her sister continued to expect that she would behave in a subservient way toward her as she had for much of their life. Mrs. Ryan began to expect more reciprocity in their relationship, which her sister did not welcome. She acknowledged that even in her old age she had changed in some ways as a person—ways that made her more independent and self-confident and also more likely to express disagreement with her sister. She expressed disagreement in muted ways and often backed off when her sister spoke sharply to her. Tension began to build in the relationship. The first major, open dispute with her sister arose after her sister's husband died 2 years earlier. "I tried to be helpful to her at first but then she kept on demanding that I do all sorts of things for her. At some point I began to say no and she was very angry. She told me that she and her husband had helped me when my husband died and now it was my turn. She said I was ungrateful. I apologized to her to make peace but I didn't really mean it. I felt she was taking advantage of me." Mrs. Ryan felt that the incident in Ireland was the endpoint of a long period of change in their relationship. "I was *not* going to return home just because my sister insisted on it. She finally realized that and now she is punishing me." The therapist pointed out that a gradual but important shift had occurred in her expectations about the relationship whereas her sister's expectations remained the same. Mrs. Ryan increasingly valued her independence. "It makes good sense that there's a problem in your relationship. Now let's try to figure out what you can do to try to mend things with your sister in a way that acknowledges her concerns as well as your own," commented the therapist. "Yes, I'd like to do that but I need a map," Mrs. Ryan replied. The therapist said, "So, let's spend the next few weeks mapping out your strategy." Mrs. Ryan looked relieved.

Session 8. The therapist again conducted the HRSD. Mrs. Ryan obtained a score of 11, which indicated *mild depression*. She was pleased that her score had decreased and acknowledged that she was feeling much better—less depressed and less anxious with better sleep and a slow return of appetite. "Now what about that map?" asked Mrs. Ryan. The therapist asked where the map would lead. "I just want my sister to be more civil to me. I just hate that she won't talk to me. It's very upsetting." It was apparent that Mrs. Ryan had little experience in negotiating differences with others. Her predominant way of handling conflict was to avoid it or capitulate. She was in need of basic communication skills training. The therapist first asked what she wanted to say to her sister. "I want her to know that she has treated me very badly and I don't like it and I want her to change." The therapist pointed out that this was probably not the best way to engage her sister in a productive conversation. He also pointed out the angry tone of her voice as she made the comment. The therapist encouraged Mrs. Ryan to think of other ways of starting a conversation with her sister. She could think of none. So the therapist offered "some ideas" about what she might try. He pointed out that most people get defensive when a conversation starts with accusations of misbehavior. The therapist asked how she felt when someone started a conversation with her in that way. She acknowledged that it made her want to "fight back." The therapist engaged her in a series of role plays in which he played her sister. It was difficult for her to do this at first but slowly she began to use less critical and more conciliatory language in these role plays. At first she felt that use of conciliatory language meant that she was "giving in." The therapist helped her to understand the distinction between giving in (i.e., a failure to honestly communicate her concerns) and having a dialogue about issues of concerns (i.e., both parties' concerns are acknowledged and respectfully communicated).

Session 9. Mrs. Ryan came with upsetting news. Her younger brother who had suffered from medical problems for many years had died. Her brother had been the sibling who was most distressed about the schism between his sisters. "He would have wanted us to make up." At the funeral Mrs. Ryan said that her sister was a little warmer to her than she had been. She said that her brother's death might be an opportunity for a reconciliation with her sister. "We're all getting on in our years." Mrs. Ryan and therapist continued to role-play a possible conversation with her sister and she demonstrated an improved ability to simulate a conversation with her sister that was more likely to open a dialogue with her. She said that she felt ready to talk to her sister in the coming week.

Session 10. The next week Mrs. Ryan complained that she was more depressed. The therapist inquired about what had happened in the prior week. She said that she saw her sister at a church social event and that "she was as cold as ever." She felt discouraged and hopeless that things could change. The therapist pointed out the connection between this event and her mood. He also reiterated that depression makes it more likely that people will feel hopeless. She said that she had thought out her plan to talk with her sister and concluded that she could not meet with her sister and talk to her. "I will get tongue tied and forget everything that we talked about and then she will just put me down. I'm not like you. You can think of the right thing to say." Mrs. Ryan and the therapist explored different ways in which she could communicate with her sister that felt comfortable, including using another family member as an intermediary or writing a letter to her sister. "Maybe if you write down the things that we've talked about, that would help," commented Mrs. Ryan. Mrs. Ryan concluded that she could speak with her sister if she had her "map" in hand but acknowledged the awkwardness of looking at a piece of paper, trying to recall what she wanted to say, while meeting with her sister. She decided that she would be able to talk to her sister on the telephone if she had a list of things she wanted to say she could refer to during the conversation.

Sessions 11 and 12. In the next sessions the therapist and Mrs. Ryan wrote out a series of things she could say to her sister. The first items were introductory comments that could engage her sister in a discussion of their dispute, such as "You know, our brother would have wanted us to be better sisters to each other. I would like to do that," "I know that both of us are hurt and upset about what has happened," and "I'd like things to be better between the two of us." After possible introductory remarks, a series of comments were written down that addressed issues in the dispute. "I know you were disappointed by what happened in Ireland. I was too. Although we had different ideas about what to do, I hope we can move on." Another series of written remarks outlined what Mrs. Ryan might say if her sister began to criticize her, such as "I know we're both upset and still I'd like for us to try improving things between us" and "I know you feel that way and I feel bad about that. I'd like to give it another try." In the next session the therapist role-played her sister as Mrs. Ryan consulted her script and responded. Mrs. Ryan said that she had her "map" now and was going to call her sister.

Session 13. The following week Mrs. Ryan said that she had called her sister and "did my best." She said that she felt awkward in the conversation but had kept herself from criticizing her sister even when her sister began to condemn her about her behavior in Ireland. She wasn't sure what was going to happen in coming weeks but hoped for the best.

Termination

Session 14. Mrs. Ryan said that she had seen her sister at the church social gathering in the prior week and that though she was not as warm to her as she had been in prior years, she was "more civil." Mrs. Ryan said she felt relieved and more hopeful that things were moving in the right direction. The therapist noted that there were two remaining sessions. "Only two? Goodness, how am I going to do this on my own?" The therapist pointed out that Mrs. Ryan had been doing things on her own with the therapist in the role of coach. She worried that she would become depressed again. The therapist also pointed out that it was normal that as therapy ended that people felt nervous about its end—but that this was not the return of depression. She said that she was sad that things would end and acknowledged that she had been skeptical that psychotherapy could be helpful. The therapist said, "It's also natural that you would feel sad. We've talked about some very important and personal things during a time that you've suffered from a depressive illness."

Session 15. Mrs. Ryan said that she had seen her sister at a family gathering and that her siblings noted that she and her sister were more hospitable to each other. "They said my dead brother would be proud of us." The therapist continued to inquire about Mrs. Ryan's feelings about terminating psychotherapy and she expressed more confidence that she could handle things on her own.

Session 16. In the final session, the therapist again conducted the HRSD, on which Mrs. Ryan scored 4, in the *nondepressed* range. She said she appreciated the therapist's help and commented, "I couldn't have done it without you." The therapist told Mrs. Ryan she couldn't have done it without herself. The therapist reviewed the course of treatment with an emphasis on the active role she had taken. "You started therapy with a major depression that followed a major dispute with your sister. You first agreed to take antidepressant medication. You were initially reluctant to come for psychotherapy but you did. You were willing to talk about difficult things, including the role that you had in the dispute with your sister. You learned new ways to communicate with your sister and had the courage to have a conversation with your sister armed with your "map." Although things aren't the way they used to be, you've told me that you wanted things to change so that you had a real voice in your relationship with your sister. And now you are no longer in a major depression and have almost no depression-related symptoms."

Case Commentary

This case illustrates how nonreciprocal role expectations led to this dispute. In Mrs. Ryan's case, the seed of the dispute was a shift in expectations about her historical relationship with her sister (prompted by her increasing independence following death of her husband). By moving the discussion from Mrs. Ryan's criticism of her sister's character to an understanding of a clash of expectations, Mrs. Ryan was better able to accept the notion that she could engage her sister in productive discussion of their interpersonal issues without seeing relationship negotiation as capitulation. By pointing out an interpersonal parallel between the way she historically interacted with her sister, her husband, and others (i.e., taking a subordinate role), she could gain a broader understanding of how she interacted with other people. Communication analysis and role play were critical in helping Mrs. Ryan develop better skills in handling the problem with her sister. Though Mrs. Ryan finally decided that she could not have a face-to-face discussion with her sister, she used a written script that aided her in having a telephone conversation with her sister. Although at the end of therapy the relationship was far from ideal, Mrs. Ryan's efforts to communicate with her sister were empowering and seemed to have led to the elimination of depressive symptoms. With her newly found sense of independence, Mrs. Ryan wanted a different relationship with her sister. Communication-related techniques were used throughout the middle phase. There was no guarantee that her sister wanted the same thing. What Mrs. Ryan was able to accomplish, however, was to open a dialogue with her sister in which there was a lowering of the interpersonal tension between them and the possibility of further dialogue.

CASE EXAMPLE: MARIA HERNANDEZ

Mrs. Hernandez was a married 69-year-old Puerto Rican woman and a retired executive secretary. The onset of depressive symptoms began several months prior to evaluation at the geriatric clinic at which time she was diagnosed with adjustment disorder with depressed mood and partner relational problem. She had an HRSD score of 16, which indicated a *mild* to *moderate depression*. She likely had had at least one episode of major depression in the past. The depressive symptoms followed an exacerbation of chronic marital problems and the initiation of an outside romantic relationship with a man. She was prescribed an SSRI antidepressant by the psychiatrist who had evaluated her. She had a history of cardiac problems and in the prior year had valve replacement surgery. Mrs. Hernandez was prescribed several medications for her cardiac condition. During the interpersonal inventory, Mrs. Hernandez indicated that she had long-standing problems with her husband that included many episodes of verbal and physical abuse over their entire marriage. Her husband had been arrested on several occasions after she called police following physical abuse. She currently had an order of protection against her husband but continued to live with him. On the way home from a medical appointment a few months after cardiac surgery, her husband had thrown her out of a moving car following a dispute. She was bruised but unharmed. In recent months she had begun a romantic relationship with Carlos, a member of her church. As she considered leaving her husband for a relationship with Carlos, she became increasingly guilty, "confused," and depressed. Mrs. Hernandez had two sons who lived nearby. She did not have good relations with either son, one of whom was a substance abuser. However, she felt very close to her daughter who lived in Puerto Rico, and with whom she had regular telephone contact and twice-yearly visits. She was raised in Puerto Rico and characterized her father as a controlling and unreasonable man. She thought her mother had done a reasonably good job of raising her but felt that she did not protect her from her father's frequent verbal outbursts. In adult life her mother told her that she had been physically abused by Mrs. Hernandez' father but she would not leave him because "once married, always married." Both her parents were deceased. On coming to the mainland United States she enrolled in college and subsequently had a successful career. She had good relationships with coworkers. After she married, her husband discouraged friendships and often was suspicious she was having extramarital affairs. Nonetheless, she had several friendships, many of them with people she met through her church.

Intermediate Sessions

Session 4. The therapist reviewed again the diagnosis of adjustment disorder, explaining that it was a psychiatric condition which in her case included depressive symptoms following a stressful life event. Mrs. Hernandez said that she was feeling better because she had decided to leave her husband and move to Puerto Rico with Carlos. Both she and her husband had known Carlos through their church. In recent months she responded to Carlos' invitation to spend time alone with him, which led to sexual intimacy. Carlos told her that she was "too good" for her husband and that it was wrong for her husband to verbally and physically abuse her. She felt protected by Carlos and imagined a life together with him. Within the IPT framework it appeared that Mrs. Hernandez was moving toward dissolution of her relationship. The therapist asked her if she had considered leaving her husband in prior years. It appeared that, in fact, she had considered this option numerous times and had had several prior affairs with men. When asked why it was more likely she would end the relationship with her husband now, she cited her age and failing health. "I have a right to some happiness in my life." The therapist felt that it was important to work with Mrs. Hernandez around clarification of past and current issues in her relationship with her husband and how their expectations and values differed. Mrs. Hernandez was not convinced that this was necessary because her decision to leave her husband was firm.

Session 5. At the beginning of the next session Mrs. Hernandez said that she was feeling more depressed. The therapist inquired about the events of the week and she said she had had an argument with her husband. She had chest pains during the night and asked her husband to take her to the hospital. "He refused and I had to call the ambulance myself. Can you believe that?" Although medical personnel at the emergency room did not feel her condition was serious enough to warrant hospitalization, she was angry that her husband would not help her. Later in the week her son with substance abuse problems came for a visit and requested money. "Like he always does, he threatened me. I told him I had given him enough money. I did give him a little money so he would leave." Carlos had been away that week visiting his adult children. She called her daughter who expressed frustration over her mother's inability to set limits with her brother and chronic ambivalence over whether she should leave her husband.

Session 6. Mrs. Hernandez said she was feeling less depressed. Her husband had been especially attentive to her during the week and had taken her to several medical appointments. They also had satisfying sexual relations. She wondered whether, in fact, she would leave her husband for Carlos. The therapist said that clearly Mrs. Hernandez had mixed feelings about what to do and said it would be helpful to gain a better understanding of the satisfying and unsatisfying aspects of her relationship with her husband. "When I met him he was a real gentleman. He was older than me. I felt like a little girl in the big city of New York. He seemed to know so much. I had left Puerto Rico to get away from my father and then I met someone who I felt would protect me." "Did he do that?" asked the therapist. "At first, but after a year or so he began to tell me what I could do and not do. I remember early in our marriage at a street fair he wanted to go home and I said no. He slapped me in front of a whole group of people and dragged me down the street." Mrs. Hernandez chronicled a long history of periodic physical and verbal abuse by her husband, family court appearances, mandated anger management classes for her husband, support groups for survivors of domestic abuse for her, and multiple orders of protection. "Why did you choose to remain with him?" asked the therapist. "Because I thought he could change. After he would hurt me he would be so nice and we had very good sex. Each time, I thought, it would be different." During the early years of her marriage Mrs. Hernandez finished college and had a series of jobs as an executive secretary. She felt that her husband tolerated this independence because she made a very good income that afforded them a solid middle-class life.

Session 7. Mrs. Hernandez said that she was again convinced that she should leave her husband. Carlos had returned. He was angry at her husband for failing to take her to the hospital and affirmed that he would never act that way toward her. "He wanted to go over and hit my husband but I told him that would only make things worse." They began to make plans for a move to Puerto Rico. The therapist encouraged Mrs. Hernandez to discuss further issues in the relationship with her husband. "He expects me to be that scared little girl who came to the big city and who needed to be taken care of. Well, I'm not that little girl any more. I'm a successful independent woman who can live her own life. I don't need anyone to tell me what to do." Despite her protest, at this point the therapist was clearly aware of Mrs. Hernandez' confusion and ambivalence about her relationship with her husband and felt that further exploration and clarification of her own thoughts and feelings about the relationship would be helpful.

Session 8. The therapist completed the HRSD at the beginning of the session. Mrs. Hernandez' score was 18 (*moderate depression*), which was higher than upon his entry into the clinic. Change in depressive symptoms was discussed with her. She mentioned that she had seen the psychiatrist earlier in the week. The psychiatrist also noted the increase in symptoms and raised the antidepressant medication. In the previous week she had had a major dispute with Carlos. Her husband had been monitoring her cell phone bill and noted frequent calls to Carlos. He called Carlos and accused him of having an affair with his wife, which Carlos denied. When Mrs. Hernandez met with Carlos he told her that it might be best to see each other less often. "I was so angry at him. What a coward! He was afraid that my husband would have a fight with him." Mrs. Hernandez told Carlos she was ending the relationship. "My husband told me that he thought I was having a relationship with Carlos but I told him that he was wrong. I said Carlos and I were friends. But I told him that if he was upset about my friendship with Carlos I would see him only at church services."

Session 9. The therapist persisted in trying to better understand the expectations and values that underlay her relationship with her husband. Clearly the theme of being protected was central to the relationship dynamic. She struggled with being independent and yet she evidenced a strong pull to dependence even on a man who physically abused her. "Mrs. Hernandez, it seems that there's a part of you who is very independent and yet another part of you who feels that she needs to be protected. From what?" She returned to a discussion of her sense of vulnerability upon arrival in New York City from Puerto Rico upon fleeing her father's many temper outbursts. Wondering whether she had failed to reveal physical abuse by her father, the therapist asked her. She said no but referred to "other things that happened when I was growing up." Despite Mrs. Hernandez' reluctance to discuss this topic, the therapist continued. Slowly and tearfully she revealed that she had been sexually abused by an uncle as a child. When she told her father of the abuse he slapped her and said that she was making things up. Her father likely said something to the uncle and the abuse stopped, yet things were never the same. "He didn't believe me and I couldn't trust him." Mrs. Hernandez said that she had once revealed the history of sexual abuse in a group for battered women and was surprised that other women in the group had a similar history.

Session 10. Mrs. Hernandez said that she was feeling less depressed. It had been hard for her to speak of her early childhood sexual abuse but she felt relieved to have told it. She had seen Carlos at church but they didn't say anything to each other and she felt convinced that the affair was ended. Her husband seemed to be kinder to her in the past week but she felt it was only a matter of time before he lost his temper. "If I understand you correctly, Mrs. Hernandez, a major problem in your relationship with your husband is that he expects you to act like you did early in your relationship—that is, pretty much do what he tells you to do. You have expected him to protect you from being hurt or harmed—like you had been as a child. Has he done that?" She said that in some ways he had been a good husband: a reasonably good provider, a satisfying sexual partner, an adequate father to their children. But what confused her was that though she looked to him for protection, he was in fact the one who hurt her most. "What do you think you most need protection from now?" asked the therapist. "I'm scared about my health. The doctor said it will likely get worse and that I will need more and more help." "Do you feel you can rely on your husband for help for current future health problems?" She shook her head and quietly said no. She recounted the trauma of being thrown out of the car shortly after heart surgery. She recalled her husband's refusal to take her to the emergency room when she was having chest pains. She said he encouraged her to take less medication than the doctor had prescribed to save money. "He helps me at times, but I just don't think I can rely on him if I get sicker."

Session 11. Mrs. Hernandez continued to be less depressed yet she did not know what to do about her relationship with her husband. The therapist encouraged her to discuss different options. She did not think that things could continue as they had. The relationship with Carlos as well as her plan to have a life with him had ended. She considered the possibility of divorcing her husband but the voice of her mother—"once married, always married"—and her religious faith made that difficult to consider. Further, divorce would leave both her and her husband in difficult economic circumstances. She considered a temporary separation but concluded that this would not solve anything. She said that any plan would have to take into account her deteriorating health. "Is there someone you could rely on if you had further health problems?" asked the therapist. "Yes, my daughter." Mrs. Hernandez said that her daughter had encouraged her and Mr. Hernandez to move to Puerto Rico. The idea of returning to her home appealed to Mrs. Hernandez but not to her husband, as he was not originally from the island. "But maybe I could move there alone and leave him here. I'll think about that."

Session 12. On the next visit, Mrs. Hernandez said that she had broached the topic of moving to Puerto Rico with her husband. He said that he did not want to move to Puerto Rico. She said that she missed her daughter and wanted to spend more time with her and her grandchildren. "He told me 'you can go, but I'm staying in New York.'" They talked on and off throughout the week about Puerto Rico and by the end of the week she proposed to him that she would spend much of the year with her daughter, returning occasionally to visit him in New York, and that he would make occasional visits to her in Puerto Rico. "I was so surprised but he thought that was a good idea." Mrs. Hernandez said that her husband was probably happy to be free of responsibility for attending to her health problems, "have the house to himself," and have less conflict with her. "And what about your daughter?" asked the therapist. Mrs. Hernandez said that her daughter welcomed the idea and was relieved that her mother finally had made a decision about what to do about the unhappy marriage.

Session 13. Mrs. Hernandez seemed especially hopeful. Plans for moving to Puerto Rico continued to be made. She thought that she could likely afford to build a house in Puerto Rico near her daughter's home. Her daughter encouraged her to come for a visit in the near future to meet with a contractor. Although her husband seemed reluctant to agree to building a house in Puerto Rico, he said he would think about it. The therapist encouraged Mrs. Hernandez to think about the practical issues associated with such a move and how she might problem-solve them. He explored with her any ambivalence about making such a move. She said that she would miss the excitement of New York, her friends at the church, and the generally satisfying sexual relationship with her husband. On the whole, however, she felt firm in her decision.

Termination

Session 14. The session was delayed because Mrs. Hernandez decided to take a trip to Puerto Rico. During the visit she met with a contractor whom she did not like but she found a piece of land near her daughter's home where she hoped she could build a house. Her husband was still reluctant to have a house built in Puerto Rico but her daughter was trying to persuade him. The therapist reminded the client that two sessions remained. She said that she had forgotten that therapy would be ending so soon and expressed concern that if there were further problems with her husband that she would have no one to talk to about them. Mrs. Hernandez felt nervous about ending therapy and sad that she would not have regular sessions with the therapist in the future. The therapist encouraged her to talk about her feelings of ending. She said that it was especially hard because she had learned to trust the therapist—enough to talk about early-childhood sexual abuse.

Session 15. Discussion continued about termination and practical issues associated with her anticipated move to Puerto Rico. An incident in the prior week had occurred in which her husband acted aggressively toward her but did not hurt her. "That made me even more certain I want to move."

Session 16. The therapist conducted the HRSD, on which the client had a score of 4. "Mrs. Hernandez, you no longer meet criteria for an adjustment disorder and have a score of 4 on the rating scale, which is in the nondepressed range." "You have helped me so much, doctor," she replied. The therapist summed up, "You have accomplished so much during the weeks that we have met together. You were depressed and took medication to help that. You came here each week to try to figure out what to do about your relationship with your husband and with Carlos. You decided to end the relationship with Carlos. You thought long and hard about the long-standing problems in your relationship with your husband and differences of expectations that were confusing for you. You examined different options and came up with one that works for you. You negotiated with your husband and are now actively making plans to change your life so that you can hopefully spend the remaining years with less conflict and have a more reliable person to help you if you have further health concerns." Mrs. Hernandez asked if sessions could continue until she moved to Puerto Rico. The therapist agreed that would be useful. They continued to see each other twice monthly, then once monthly until Mrs. Hernandez moved. The therapist connected Mrs. Hernandez to mental health resources in Puerto Rico.

Case Commentary

Although IPT for the treatment of major depression has been formally adapted for the treatment of a variety of conditions, no studies of its usefulness in adjustment disorder exist. In clinical practice, we have found it to be a useful modality with older adults. Because adjustment disorder is not accompanied by the vegetative symptoms or marked impairment in daily functioning usually evident in major depression, we put less emphasis on adjustment disorder as a medical illness than we do with major depression. We continue to remind the client that adjustment disorder is a psychiatric condition with significant symptoms of depression (and as may be the case, anxiety) that makes it more difficult to function.

Mrs. Hernandez' case was a troubling one. She had a long history of domestic abuse. As she developed more health problems she felt increasingly vulnerable. It was, of course, shocking to learn that she had been thrown out of an automobile by her husband shortly after heart surgery. The stage of her dispute vacillated among renegotiation, impasse, and dissolution. Ambivalence about one's relationship with a spouse and remaining in circumstances in which a person is being physically harmed are common issues for abused spouses. Use of IPT's strategy of focusing on nonreciprocal role expectations was especially helpful to Mrs. Hernandez in clarifying why she remained with her husband. Use of this strategy included a reckoning with the role of early-childhood abuse in shaping her sense of vulnerability and need for protection and how expectations about these issues were brought forward into adult life and marriage. From an adult development and aging perspective, the onset of health problems in later life raised another set of concerns about physical vulnerability and a reckoning that her husband could not be relied on to help her. Therapy provided an opportunity to take stock of her life, generate options, balance values and practical concerns in choosing an option, and begin to make efforts to implement the option. In the end she chose not to dissolve her marriage but make major changes to it so that she and her husband had minimal contact. This active and empowering decision was associated with a significant decrease in depressive symptoms. Although therapists may feel pessimistic that long-standing interpersonal problems in older adults are amenable to change, this and other cases in our clinical work are evidence that change is possible. Nonetheless, a life history of physical abuse by her husband very likely left Mrs. Hernandez with psychological and emotional trauma that would benefit by ongoing mental health care (Wolkenstein & Sterman, 1998).

CONCLUDING COMMENTARY

Among our older IPT clients, interpersonal role disputes are common as the primary focus of psychotherapy or as a secondary area. Despite the stereotypical characterization of older adults as rigid and unable to change, we find many older clients willing to try new ways to negotiate new or long-standing interpersonal problems. Older adults seen in therapy are often motivated by the hope of reducing emotional distress tied to the dispute and a willingness to consider other ways of handling the dispute. The reality of failing health or anticipation of failing health may also motivate some older adults to try to mend relationships on which they will increasingly rely for practical and emotional support. What has impressed us is that building fairly basic communication skills with older clients can have substantive results. As noted in chapter 2 (this volume), this generation of older adults is generally less familiar with psychological and interpersonal concepts than are cohorts of younger individuals who have been raised in a more psychologically minded era. Yet living many years has taught most older adults that there usually are two sides to every dispute and that peace—in which the views of both parties are acknowledged—is better than war.

8

ROLE TRANSITIONS

As noted in chapters 2 and 4 (this volume), the transitional nature of late life has long been of concern to gerontologists. Social gerontologists were especially concerned that the loss of social roles—notably those of parent and worker—decreased social opportunities and increased the likelihood that old age would be without norms and values (Rosow, 1967). The lack of norms and values puts older adults at greater risk for depleted morale, decreased life satisfaction, and depression. Studies have, however, documented that older adults generally adapt to late-life role transitions and maintain emotional well-being. Nonetheless, some older adults encounter substantive difficulties with late-life role transitions. More recent gerontological research has emphasized that the acquisition of new roles in late life may be equally or more stressful than role loss (Schulz, O'Brien, Bookwala, & Fleissner, 1995). Health-related role acquisitions include transitioning into the role of a person with health problems or the role of caregiver for a spouse or partner with health problems. Some older adults find themselves transitioning into parenting roles to care for grandchildren when their own children, for one or more reasons, are unable to fulfill parenting obligations (Pruchno, 1999). Life transitions are not unique to late life and, in fact, adulthood is a series of building new life structures and periods of transitions between them (Levinson, 1986) as well as a changing sense of "possible selves" (Markus & Nurius,

1986). These transitional periods are the most stressful times in people's lives as people need to emotionally reckon with the life that has been lived, the demands of the new life era, and the challenges of rebuilding a life structure.

In geriatric clinical practice, health-related role transitions are the type of transition most frequently encountered. The modal case is that of an older woman who begins caring for a husband with dementia. Research has documented that care for a person with dementia is enormously stressful and prolonged and often results in negative mental and physical health consequences for the caregiver (Aneshensel, Pearlin, Mullan, Zarit, & Whitlatch, 1995; Schulz et al., 1990). Other caregiving scenarios include care for a spouse with physical infirmities or mental health problems. Less common are cases in which older clients are confronted with responsibilities for care of a seriously ill child or sibling. In the case of a spouse with dementia, acquisition of the caregiving role is also accompanied by loss of the marital role as it had been known. Despite gerontological concerns about the adverse emotional impact of the loss of roles of parent or worker, in clinical practice, only occasionally are retirement or "empty nest" central issues. Research studies have consistently documented that most individuals make a relatively smooth transition into retirement and that the empty-nest syndrome is not a common phenomenon (Crowley, Hayslip, & Hobdy, 2003).

GOALS AND STRATEGIES OF IPT FOR ROLE TRANSITIONS

Goals are threefold: mourning and acceptance of the loss of the old role; helping the patient to regard the new role as more positive; and restoring self-esteem by developing a sense of mastery regarding demands of the new role (see Exhibit 8.1). For most individuals a change in the structure of life is emotionally dislocating. The familiarity and predictability of an established pattern of living—as sociologists would argue (e.g., Rosow, 1967), mediated through one or several roles—can be comforting. The way one views one's self, other, and world is interwoven with existing roles. Loss of the role or roles is commonly associated with feelings of sadness. In interpersonal psychotherapy (IPT), an explicit acknowledgment of loss is accompanied by working through associated feelings. Therapeutic facilitation of the goal of helping the client to regard the new role as more positive helps to shift the client's perspective that role change can be regarded only as loss to a view that the new role may have opportunities that had not been considered.

Taking this affirmative therapeutic stance can be challenging for novice therapists or those who have not worked with older adults. Further, it may be difficult for those with little geriatric experience to understand that, for example, there can be rewards in caring for someone who is ill. Health problems cannot be welcomed events, yet even adversity has within it the

EXHIBIT 8.1
Outline of Interpersonal Psychotherapy for Major Depression

C. Role Transitions
1. Goals
   a. Mourning and acceptance of the loss of the old role.
   b. Help the patient to regard the new role as more positive.
   c. Restore self-esteem by developing a sense of mastery regarding demands of new role.
2. Strategies
   a. Review depressive symptoms.
   b. Relate depressive symptoms to difficulty in coping with some recent life change.
   c. Review positive and negative aspects of old and new roles.
   d. Explore feelings about what is lost.
   e. Explore feelings about the change itself.
   f. Explore opportunities in new role.
   g. Realistically evaluate what is lost.
   h. Encourage appropriate release of affect.
   i. Encourage development of social support system and of new skills called for in new role.

Note. From *Comprehensive Guide to Interpersonal Psychotherapy* (pp. 23–24), by M. M. Weissman, J. C. Markowitz, and G. L. Klerman, 2000, New York: Basic Books. Copyright 2000 by Basic Books. Reprinted with permission.

possibility for personal satisfaction and growth. We are not culturally well prepared to regard health-related problems as having within them potentially positive attributes. As part of a research study, Clougherty conducted IPT with HIV-positive individuals with depression, most of whom were gay men (Markowitz et al., 1999). It was notable that these clients generally were able to shift their view of HIV as a death sentence in early life to a perspective that HIV presented opportunities for cultivating more meaningful relationships with others, formulating a new or enhanced philosophy of life, and developing new activities and interests. At the end of therapy they also evidenced a significant reduction in depressive symptoms. The study was conducted prior to the advent of life-prolonging HIV medications, at a time when most of those infected could realistically expect to die. The IPT therapist is similarly challenged to develop an affirmative stance about possibilities for a meaningful life for the client even within the constraints of health-related role change.

The third goal—restoration of self-esteem by enhancing mastery of the new role—involves the client's reckoning with the parameters of the new role and the acquisition of skills to better fulfill the role. Transition into health-related problems may confront the individual with a new set of demands which he or she may not feel capable of handling. We sometimes compare health-related role transitions with starting a new job for which there is a steep learning curve. For instance, an older client seen in clinical practice was initially overwhelmed with the onset of diabetes. As she became more compliant with dietary restrictions, glucose monitoring, and taking prescribed medications, depressive symptoms abated. Though she regretted that she had to contend with medical problems, within the parameters of that reality, she felt increasingly empowered by her health-promoting behaviors. In the gerontology caregiver literature, sense of mastery about handling caregiving-related problems has been tied to better caregiver emotional well-being (Aneshensel et al., 1995). For example, dementia caregivers sometimes feel defeated that their efforts to manage behavioral problems often evident in dementia do not seem to work. For many caregivers, the job of caring for a relative with dementia will be the most complex task they have ever undertaken as it requires a host of skills that must be learned.

Strategies 2a and 2b: Review depressive symptoms. Relate depressive symptoms to difficulty in coping with some recent life change. As in all the IPT problem areas, depression and depression-related symptoms are reviewed on a regular basis. The onset of symptoms was tied to the life change in the initial sessions, but clients sometimes lose sight of this connection. This connection bears repeating during the middle sessions.

Strategy 2c: Review positive and negative aspects of old and new roles. The client may be inclined to view life before the new role in ways that emphasize only positive aspects. For example, an older client who stopped working because of health problems spoke only of the pleasure she had derived from work. She recounted the satisfying aspects of her relationship with coworkers, the gratifying challenge of dealing with the many and varied aspects of her job, and feeling of loyalty to the company for which she worked. This focus accentuated the loss that she felt on leaving her job. The therapist encouraged her to speak in more detail about her work life including those days when work was not as enjoyable as usual or when things "didn't go so well." She conceded that she didn't like several of her coworkers, felt overwhelmed at times by too many responsibilities, and spent less time with friends and family than she had wished because she often had to work late. The end of her work life had, in fact, brought opportunity to spend more time with her family, sleep late, and not contend with work-related stress. Use of this therapeutic strategy helped her to take a more balanced view of work and with it a fuller reckoning of the positive and negative aspects of her life as a person with health-related problems.

As noted earlier, it may be initially hard for the client (as well as the novice therapist) to see positive aspects of health-related roles. For example, early research on stresses of dementia caregiving focused chiefly on the problems faced by family caregivers. Later research documented that many family caregivers could delineate positive aspects of their roles, including improvement in some aspects of the relationship with the care receiver, an enhanced sense of mastery in the caregiving role, greater family solidarity, and satisfaction that they had "done the right thing" in caring for the impaired relative (Beach, Schulz, Yee, & Jackson, 2000). Although problems typically outnumber rewards for most caregivers, it is important not to lose sight of the fact that helping others can bring important rewards. In IPT, the therapist will therefore encourage an accounting of the many dimensions of the new role to help the client to have a fuller understanding of the pluses and minuses of the new role. Older adults transitioning into parenting roles for grandchildren (Pruchno, 1999) often speak of the loss or reduction of recreational and social interests but also of the opportunity to establish a close relationship with the grandchild along with the conviction that they have fulfilled larger family obligations.

Strategy 2d: Explore feelings about what is lost and **Strategy 2e:** Explore feelings about the change itself. Strategies 2d and 2e are related to Strategy 2c (Review positive and negative aspects of old and new roles). Facilitation of feelings not only results in a therapeutic release of painful affect but also provides the client with a fuller understanding of the emotional impact of the life change. Gradual, therapist-guided work in this area helps the client to grieve the life role that has been altered and come to terms with current life circumstances. These strategies have parallels with some of those used in IPT's grief problem area as they help the client to emotionally process the loss—albeit loss tied to a web of role-related relationships, activities, and a way of life. Just as moving on from the death of a significant other often requires emotional processing of the loss, so does a transition from one role to another (Levinson, 1986). One older IPT client who was physically disabled from arthritis brought in a picture of herself as a young woman waving to the camera while waterskiing. She laughed and cried as she recounted events surrounding the vacation during which the picture was taken. She pointed to the three-prong cane which she now used to walk and said that the cane now pulled her along. She said that she hated the fact that she was disabled and wished that she were again that young woman on skis. "Oh, those were the days." She said that she knew that wasn't realistic but "that's the way I feel." With that emotional reckoning she was better able to maximize independence within the parameters of her disability.

Strategy 2f: Explore opportunities in the new role. This strategy also may be implemented in tandem with Strategy 2c in which there is review of positive and negative aspects of the old and new role. Opportunities may include freedom from former role-related demands and options to pursue interests or relationships that previously had not been possible in the old role. One client was treated with IPT for depression following the onset of blindness. She was devastated by her loss because she had been a devoted and lifelong reader. "It's the worst possible thing that could happen to me." Other reading options were reviewed with her and she eventually began to listen to books-on-tape. Because family members now took care of home-making responsibilities for which she had been previously responsible, she actually had more hours each week to devote to books.

Strategy 2g: Realistically evaluate what is lost. Again, this strategy can be used in tandem with Strategy 2c (Review positive and negative aspects of old and new roles). An honest reckoning of what has been lost in transition from one role to another facilitates expression of affect, identification of what was most important in the prior role, and review of options for gaining via the new role some aspects of what had been lost.

Strategy 2h: Encourage appropriate release of affect. Encouragement of appropriate affect may take place in conjunction with all of the above strategies. The therapist's encouragement of the client to speak in a detailed way about issues of concern is more likely to elicit affect than a global recount. The client's stories are occasionally flooded with affect in a session. If this happens, the therapist may want to circumscribe the discussion to help calm the client and return to the issue in the next session.

Strategy 2i: Encourage development of social supports and of new skills called for in the new role. New roles call for new skills and often clients do not feel that they possess some or all of them. A client with medical problems may not know how to effectively negotiate with service providers to get what he or she wants. The therapist begins the discussion with an exploration of existing options and may encourage the client to pursue the development of needed skills. For clients who have trouble generating options, the therapist may offer suggestions. For dementia caregivers, learning multiple skill sets is often needed. Skills may include ways to calm an agitated person, handle repetitive questioning, safeguard the person from behaviors that may be dangerous, hire and manage home health aides, and facilitate social or recreational engagements for the person. Because so many challenges usually are associated with dementia care, the caregiver may feel overwhelmed and pessimistic that anything can be done. It is often helpful to break down caregiving responsibilities into discreet tasks and their associated skills. The therapist can then encourage the client to try out specific skills. Success or lack of success in implementing skills can then be reviewed in the subsequent sessions.

New roles also require reckoning with the expansion or refashioning of existing social supports. Medically ill individuals may not want to call on friends or family for assistance. The therapist should encourage the client to identify potential sources of help and support. Reluctance to ask for assistance may be addressed by exploring the reasons for that reluctance and, as needed, role-playing ways to request help. Caregivers of infirm older adults also are often reticent to ask family or service providers for help even when it is available. For example, research studies have found that some caregivers are reluctant to use respite services even when they are affordable and available (Cox, 1997). Common concerns that feed this reluctance included a conviction that the person with dementia can be adequately cared for only by the caregiver, fear of burdening others, anxiety that something terrible will happen if the caregiver is not present, and an uneasiness about spending resources to hire home health aides for fear the money won't last. A related issue is that the caregiving role often becomes the only focus of the caregiver's life. Sociologists have characterized this phenomenon as *role engulfment* (i.e., the caregiver role totally takes over the individual's life to the exclusion of other roles and social and recreational activities that were previously enjoyed; Aneshensel et al., 1995). Psychodynamic psychologists have dubbed this phenomenon *caregiver symbiosis* (i.e., interpersonal boundaries between caregiver and relative begin to disappear as the caregiver's identity and well-being become inextricably tied to that of the impaired relative; Rose & DelMaestro, 1990). The therapist works with the client to realistically evaluate these concerns. Also, the therapist helps the client to review options for acquiring support, ways to engage other people, and activities that promote emotional well-being.

CONTINUATION OF THE CASE OF MAY BARTON

To recap: Mrs. Barton is a 74-year-old, married woman whose husband Peter had a stroke 3 years earlier that left him with physical disabilities. Six months prior to her starting IPT he had another stroke that left him with cognitive impairment, following which Mrs. Barton developed a major depression. She had had one and possibly two prior episodes of major depression. She had difficulty accepting that her husband had dementia, dealing with her husband's changed behavior, and managing the home health aide.

Intermediate Sessions

Sessions 4 and 5. Mrs. Barton complained that her home was "a mess" and said she could not motivate herself to care for her home. She was disappointed with how the home health aide cared for the house and how she herself couldn't accomplish what she felt she should. "What's wrong with me?" The therapist reiterated that major depression made it much more difficult to function and that, for the time being, she would be wise to reduce her usual level of home responsibilities until she was feeling less depressed. Focusing on concerns related to the aide, the therapist reviewed how she communicated expectations to the aide about care of her husband and care of their home. "I told her when she first came what needed to be done and now she doesn't do everything I asked." It became apparent during exploration of this issue that Mrs. Barton avoided communicating concerns to the aide under the assumption that the aide would remember her original instructions. She also feared a confrontation with the aide and wondered whether the aide might treat her husband less kindly if her concerns were brought to the aide's attention. Mrs. Barton noted that until her husband's illness no one had ever worked for her, as she had been a homemaker her entire life. The therapist pointed out that Mrs. Barton was now an employer and that part of that role was managing the aide. The therapist encouraged the client to think of different options to communicate expectations to the aide. She said that she might call the agency that provided the aide and complain or perhaps give the aide a daily list of tasks that needed to be completed.

Session 6. Mrs. Barton said she was feeling more depressed. The aide had arrived late several times in the past week and continued to perform household responsibilities in a way that disappointed her. The therapist again encouraged Mrs. Barton to review the options that had been generated in the prior week. She said that she would think about what to do. The therapist noted that depressive symptoms had increased and that the increase appeared tied to problems with the aide. "I really must do something," commented Mrs. Barton. The therapist role-played a possible conversation she might have with the aide. She struggled with how to convey her concerns to the aide. By the end of the role play she seemed to find a strategy to speak with the aide that balanced directness and diplomacy. "I appreciate the help that you are providing to my husband over the past several months. He likes you. I thought this would be a good time to talk about how things have been going. I know that you have a lot going on in your life but I'd really appreciate it if you'd make every effort to be on time. Also, maybe I wasn't as clear as I should have been about what needs to be done around the house. I've made a list of things that need to be done each day. Could we go over that together?"

Session 7. Mrs. Barton arrived at the next session smiling. She had the planned conversation with the aide and, to her surprise, the aide apologized and promised to be on time. They also went over the list of tasks that needed to be done. Nonetheless, Mrs. Barton said that she was growing increasingly frustrated with her husband's behavior. Not only did he spend much of the day watching videos, but he watched the same video over and over. "He's turning into a vegetable. It's just not right for him to sit there watching videos." The therapist inquired about what she expected from her husband. "He should read the paper or at least watch different videos." Prior to his recent stroke, Peter had been an avid newspaper reader. Since his stroke he seemed to have lost interest. "Why might that be?" asked the therapist. Mrs. Barton said that she did not know. The therapist gently encouraged her to think about the possibility that the second stroke had made him less mentally able to concentrate. "Yes, but he should try harder. When he had his first stroke the physical therapist pushed him to walk. I need to push him to read the paper, don't I?" The therapist suggested that physical disability and mental disability were different and that, in fact, her husband's second stroke had challenged her with a different set of problems that required different ways of responding to them. Mrs. Barton asked the therapist if he thought her husband should see another doctor to see if something could be done about his "problems with thinking." It appeared that her husband had not been evaluated by a neurologist recently and the therapist gave her the name of one.

Returning to concerns that her husband watched the same video over and over, the therapist asked if he appeared to enjoy the video. "Oh, yes. It's the movie *Oklahoma*. It was always his favorite." "So it seems that it's more a problem for you than him?" "He still shouldn't watch the same movie. He should watch other movies too."

Session 8. At the beginning of the eighth session the therapist again conducted the Hamilton Rating Scale for Depression (HRSD). Her score was 9 (*mild depression*), which indicated some improvement in depressive symptoms. Mrs. Barton acknowledged that she was feeling a bit better but she still felt overwhelmed by her caregiving responsibilities. Despite her conversation with the aide, the aide was late in arriving the previous week. "Did you speak with her about that?" asked the therapist. She said no but would if the aide were late again. She also complained that despite the conversation with the aide, the aide had failed to complete several tasks that were on the list that had been given to her. Mrs. Barton also said that she had made an appointment for her husband with the neurologist.

Session 9. Mrs. Barton arrived and announced, "I fired her!" She said that the aide had been late twice in the prior week and she called the agency and asked for another aide. The agency dispatched another aide whom she liked. She was satisfied with the new aide's work and was hopeful that things would work out better than with the previous aide. She also said that her husband had been seen by the neurologist. "He said the same thing that you did. He has dementia." She wondered, however, whether the neurologist might be wrong. But there was another problem. Her husband had diabetes and needed to be careful about what he ate. In the past week, she found that he had gone to the refrigerator and ate a whole cheesecake. Following that, his blood sugar was high. The therapist encouraged Mrs. Barton to think of options to restrict her husband's access to certain foods. She felt bad about doing this because "He has so little to look forward to." She finally decided that she would wrap up certain foods in the refrigerator because "you men will never go to the bother of unwrapping something in the refrigerator if you are hungry!" She also decided to put out a limited amount of fruit that her husband could snack on during the day when he was hungry.

Session 10. Mrs. Barton said she was feeling very upset. "I think my husband needs to be put on psychiatric medication." This comment was notable given Mrs. Barton's own reluctance to take antidepressant medication. Mrs. Barton explained that Peter began to make sexual comments to the new home health aide. She was mortified when she overheard him making these comments to the aide and so embarrassed that she refused to repeat the words. "I think he needs to be medicated." The therapist encouraged Mrs. Barton to provide a detailed account of when the sexual comments were more likely to happen. At first, she said they appeared to come "from nowhere" yet the discussion revealed that the comments emerged when the aide was bathing her husband and in the morning when the aide woke him up. "So the comments happen at bath time and in his bedroom. Is that correct?" "Yes. Perhaps it's the stimulation of the water or something that arouses him." "Yes, and also the fact that your husband is in a situation where he is without clothing in the presence of a young woman whom he may find attractive."

Mrs. Barton said that her husband was always one to "tease the girls" but he never was coarse. "Why do you think that is now?" asked the therapist. She answered, "Because something is broken in his brain. You know I was looking at the electrical box in our apartment the other day and saw all these wires and I thought to myself, 'It's like Peter's brain. It's like some of those wires have been cut and they can't be put back together. When he makes those comments it's like things have gone haywire and he can't control himself.'" Because the therapist felt that Mrs. Barton was ready to have a more direct discussion of the topic of dementia, he commented, "That's a very good way of putting things. That's what happens in dementia." "So what can I do about his sexual remarks?" she asked. Different options were discussed. She said that she had spoken to the aide after hearing sexual comments. The aide said that she did not take it personally and understood that her husband was a "sick man." Mrs. Barton finally decided that when the aide bathed her husband she would keep away so that if he did make sexual remarks she would not hear them. "It sounds like it's more upsetting for you than for the aide." "It is. I know he can't control himself. It's those broken wires." She also decided that she would get her husband out of bed in the morning rather than having the aide do it so as to avoid a trigger for his remarks. At the end of the session Mrs. Barton concluded by saying, "I guess he doesn't really need medication. Maybe I'm the one who needs medication to calm me down!" "You did find something that will calm you down and that is your plan for handling this situation."

Session 11. Having found a metaphor for coming to terms with her husband's dementia, she began the next session with a discussion of her marriage prior to her husband's recent stroke. She said that they had had a loving marriage. She was proud of the fact that he had been a fireman and that he had fought in World War II. She brought in a wedding picture and remarked how handsome her husband was. "He was always my tower of strength. I feel like I've lost my companion." His retirement several years ago was a welcome event because she and her husband had the opportunity to spend much more time together. "Even after his first stroke things weren't so bad because we could talk and share with each other. And now it seems like he's disappearing. Oh, he looks the same and at times he seems the same. There are glimmers of what he once was. And when I see those glimmers I feel sad and happy at the same time." She began to cry. "I'll be all right. It's just been so hard to accept what I've lost with his second stroke."

Session 12. Mrs. Barton said that she was feeling "much better." The new aide was working out well and she felt more comfortable in giving direct feedback to the aide. It still bothered her that Peter watched a limited number of videos "but I now understand that's enjoyable to him. Sometimes, however, I get tired of hearing them! So I go to our bedroom and read." She had a recent conversation with her daughter. Her daughter was relieved that Mrs. Barton had acknowledged that Peter had dementia and that she continued in psychotherapy. Her daughter also invited her and Peter for a visit. Mrs. Barton was nervous about doing this because she wasn't sure her husband would be able to handle it. However, she felt she needed a break and was pleased that her daughter said that she would take over direct care responsibilities for Peter if they visited so that her mother could have "a real vacation." Mrs. Barton returned to a recounting of her early life with Peter and brought in a family photo album which she and the therapist looked through. "He's not the man he used to be but I'm so proud that he helped so many people during his life. Did you know he helped liberate one of those concentration camps during World War II? He never wanted to talk about it much. I knew it must have been very hard for him." She was again tearful during this discussion.

Session 13. Mrs. Barton said that it had been a difficult week for her. Her arthritis had "flared up," she was in more pain, and she had more difficulties walking. She had to rely on the aide to help her. She felt a bit more depressed than she had in the prior week. Peter had made a run on the refrigerator and ate a pound of baloney that she had forgotten to wrap up and he seemed to be more confused than usual. At one point she found her husband walking out the door when the aide was out grocery shopping. "I wonder if another one of those wires was cut in his brain." The session focused on a review of options to deal with recent difficulties.

Termination

Session 14. The therapist reminded Mrs. Barton that two sessions remained. She expressed sadness over the ending of the therapy. "You've been such a good friend. Well, *friend* is not the right word. You've been someone who I could really talk to like you would with a good friend." She wondered if she would be able to handle things on her own after the end of therapy. The therapist emphasized that it was normal for clients to feel sad and a little uneasy anticipating the end of therapy. She said she understood but that it was still hard to end. She had decided to travel with Peter for a visit to her daughter's home. She was worried about how she would manage getting to the airport and getting her husband on to the plane. Different options were reviewed and Mrs. Barton decided to ask the aide for help getting to the airport. She also planned to call the airline company to arrange for a wheelchair.

Session 15. Discussion of the ending of therapy continued in this session. She said she was feeling nervous in the prior week as she thought about the end of therapy and wondered whether she was getting more depressed. A review of depressive symptoms did not indicate this and therapist reiterated that it was common that people felt this way on ending treatment. Mrs. Barton said she felt she needed ongoing support after the end of therapy. She inquired about the availability of a support group for family members caring for relatives with dementia. Such a group was available in the clinic and the therapist promised to make arrangements for her entry into the group. Further discussion centered on the planned trip to her daughter's home and problem solving of issues of concern related to the trip.

Session 16. The therapist conducted the HRSD in the final session. Mrs. Barton had a score of 3, which was in the nondepressed range. "You have a score of 3 on this scale that measures depression. A score of 3 means that you have almost no depression-related symptoms. Further, you are no longer in a major depression." Mrs. Barton expressed relief at this news and recalled her prior episode of depression, which was much more severe than the current episode. "When I began to get depressed this time I thought it was wise to get professional help so that I wouldn't get as depressed as before." "I think that was a wise decision," responded the therapist. "Although we can't say for sure, without therapy things could have gotten much worse." She replied, "Oh, I know they would have. And then what would I have done? When I was depressed before I couldn't get out of bed. Can you imagine what it would be like if both Peter and I were disabled?" Mrs. Barton again expressed some nervousness about ending therapy. The therapist remarked, "I think you're in a much better position to handle things now. When your husband had his second stroke your role changed. It changed from caring for someone with physical disability to caring for someone with both physical and mental disability. It was very hard for you to accept the fact that your husband had dementia." "That's true," said Mrs. Barton. "Remember when I looked at the electrical box and thought about those broken wires? That's when I began to accept what had happened." "I remember that. You have done so many things to deal with the problems that you've confronted in caring for your husband. You dealt with the situation with the aide who wasn't performing as you wished. You were upset about Peter's sexual remarks toward the aide but you figured out how to deal with them so that they were less upsetting to you. You worked out a way so that Peter was less likely to eat foods he shouldn't." "Yes, but remember when he ate the pound of baloney?!" "Yes, but there have been fewer problems than before."

"You've also come to terms with what you've lost since Peter's second stroke," commented the therapist. Mrs. Barton replied, "I'm still coming to terms with that. But I realize that I have a disabled husband and I'm grateful that I still have a husband. Many of my friends have lost their husbands. Although Peter has many problems, I enjoy times when we are together when I see glimmers of what he was. And I know that I have a husband whom I can be very proud of." "I think you can be very proud of yourself for all the efforts that you have made in therapy." "Yes, I'm pleased and, as you say, I think I am in a better position to handle things. I'm still learning but I'm better at it." The therapist advised Mrs. Barton that upon returning from the visit to her daughter's home she could start the weekly dementia support group. She remained in the geriatric clinic, so she asked if she could call occasionally. He said that would be fine.

Case Commentary

The three goals of IPT treatment of role transitions were addressed in this case. Mrs. Barton better came to emotional terms with the loss of the relationship she had had with her husband before the onset of his dementia. She learned to find ways to enjoy her husband despite his disability and found her caregiver role more tolerable. She also felt more capable of handling problems tied to care for her husband with an increased sense of mastery of the role. During the therapy there was a great deal of problem solving of caregiving issues and use of associated behavior change techniques. Exploration, encouragement of affect, and clarification techniques were also used primarily in the service of strategies to help Mrs. Barton emotionally contend with the fact that her husband had dementia and with the change in their relationship. She better learned to use and manage the home health aides, and at the end of therapy, she transitioned into an ongoing caregiver support group.

CASE EXAMPLE: CAL LEWIS

Mr. Lewis was a retired, widowed 66-year-old, Baptist, African American man. Clinical evaluation indicated that Mr. Lewis was experiencing major depression, moderate, single episode. His HRSD score was 22, which indicates significant depression. Mr. Lewis was in generally good health. He had hypertension and was taking an antihypertensive medication. Mr. Lewis had lost his wife 2 years earlier following a brief illness. He appeared to have coped reasonably well with the loss. He had two daughters. There was limited contact with his oldest daughter, with whom he had an estranged relationship. The estrangement was tied to problems his daughter had with drug use when she was young, at which time Mr. Lewis told his daughter to leave the home. When she was alive, Mr. Lewis's wife maintained contact with his oldest daughter, who subsequently stopped using drugs, married, and had a child. However, Mrs. Lewis had never met his grandchild because his daughter refused to see him. Mr. Lewis spoke bitterly about this. About a year ago his youngest daughter, Carrie, returned to his home shortly after she gave birth to a baby boy. Carrie returned because she was experiencing financial and practical problems as a single mother. Mr. Lewis transitioned into providing almost full-time care for the baby as his daughter worked during the day. He grew increasingly frustrated with these responsibilities. Despite the fact that they had previously had a generally good relationship, they began to have a series of angry arguments over child-care issues. Six months after Carrie's return home, Mr. Lewis began to get depressed. He then visited his internist because of weight loss and sleep problems. His internist prescribed antidepressant medication, which did not improve his condition. Eventually the internist referred him to the geriatric clinic. The clinic psychiatrist changed the antidepressant medication. During the interpersonal inventory, Mr. Lewis said he had a generally good relationship with his infirm mother who required ongoing assistance. He also had two siblings. He had limited contact with his brother, whom he characterized as "difficult to get along with." He had a better relationship with his sister although they periodically quarreled about how to divide responsibilities for care of their mother. Mr. Lewis regularly bowled with several friends from his former job. He was an active member of his church. In the initial sessions Mr. Lewis's problem areas were identified as role transition (i.e., transitioning into the role of care for his grandchild) and interpersonal role dispute (i.e., difficulties with his daughter Carrie).

Intermediate Sessions

Session 4. Mr. Lewis arrived at the session appearing quite agitated. Remarking on this, the therapist asked him how he was feeling. "I'm disgusted with my daughter. What kind of mother is she? She was supposed to take care of the baby last night but at the last minute went out with her friends. She left me having to take care of the baby and I wanted to go bowling. So I said, 'Okay, just go.' The baby wasn't feeling well and cried on and off all evening. I didn't know what to do." Mr. Lewis reluctantly acknowledged he was feeling more depressed. The therapist inquired about how childcare responsibilities had been negotiated with his daughter. "It's all on her terms." Despite several efforts to clarify this issue, Mr. Lewis was vague. He was similarly vague when the therapist shifted to a broader discussion of why and how he had agreed to invite his daughter to live with him after she had the baby. "What else should I have done?" Mr. Lewis had considerable difficulty engaging in a focused discussion and left the session as upset as he had been when the session began.

Session 5. In the next session Mr. Lewis seemed calmer. He said that his daughter had taken the baby to the pediatrician who found his grandchild had an ear infection. The baby was treated with antibiotics and was doing better and was easier to manage. He had been bowling with his friends in the previous week and enjoyed the outing. The therapist noted that his better mood seemed to be tied to the baby's improvement as well as the opportunity to spend time with his friends. The therapist then returned to the question of how he had assumed the role of care for his grandchild. He said that he felt sorry for his daughter because she was having a difficult time being a single mother. He also felt a family obligation to help out his daughter. "Did she ask you if she could return home?" asked the therapist. "No, I asked her. Sometimes I regret it, though." After the therapist pushed hard for specifics, it appeared that at the time his daughter returned home, Mr. Lewis and his daughter had not negotiated what the parameters of his responsibilities would be for care of the child. His daughter had mentioned arranging child care for the baby when she first returned home but this had not happened. He found himself responsible for much more care for the child than he assumed would be the case. He also expressed frustration over his perceived inadequacies as a parent to his grandson. "What do I know about babies? What do I know about what to do if the baby is crying? My wife always did that." He expressed regret that his wife had died because "she would have known what to do." Mr. Lewis said his wife was a good mother and had a way of handling the children that he admired, and felt that if his wife were alive the situation would be much better. Asked if he had considered discussing his concerns with his daughter, he said that he had tried but it always led to arguments. The therapist reiterated that Mr. Lewis's depression was tied to his new role as a parent and disputes with his daughter. He agreed with this observation.

Session 6. Mr. Lewis again arrived at the session appearing agitated. His daughter had criticized him in the prior week because he bought the wrong baby formula and said that he was not feeding the baby at regular enough intervals. Therein followed an angry argument with his daughter during which the baby started crying. "My daughter said, 'Do you see what you've done? You've upset the baby.' My daughter took the baby and left the house. She spent the night at a friend's house. When she returned the next day she said she was leaving and told me that she and the baby would never see me again. I told her that I was sorry and asked her to stay. She didn't say anything and things have been tense." The therapist said that his daughter's threat to leave must have been very upsetting to him especially because his oldest daughter and her child had limited contact with him. The thought of a break with both of his children must have troubled him. At this point Mr. Lewis appeared to fight back tears. The therapist encouraged him to talk about what had happened that led to the estrangement with his oldest daughter. Initially he spoke angrily about his daughter's drug use and "the life she had chosen for herself." Eventually he acknowledged that he could have handled things better with his oldest daughter and that his wife had asked him to make amends with her, which he refused to do.

Session 7. The therapist reviewed Mr. Lewis's symptoms and he seemed somewhat less depressed. He said that he had thought about what had been discussed in the prior session and acknowledged that he was regretful about what had happened with his oldest daughter. He was heartbroken that he had never seen his grandchild. The therapist inquired about whether these regrets might have had something to do with his invitation to Carrie to return home. He said that he had hoped "to get things right this time" by taking on the role as parent to his grandson. The therapist asked him what had been lost and what had been gained by assuming this new role. He said that he missed time by himself, opportunities to be with his friends, and the church involvements that he had before the baby came. "My life was more relaxed. Since my wife died I've been a little lonely too." Mr. Lewis said that what he hoped to gain by being a parent to his grandchild was to experience what he could not with his oldest daughter's child. He often enjoyed time with the baby but felt bad that he didn't know how to best handle his responsibilities. He said that though his daughter seemed to "more naturally" know what to do, she was learning how to be a parent too. He feared, however, that despite hopes that assuming a parenting role for his grandchild might lead to a closer relationship with his daughter and her son, the opposite seemed to be happening. "I just don't know what to do." The therapist said, "That's a good place to start. Let's think about your options and what you might be able to do."

Session 8. The therapist administered the HRSD on which Mr. Lewis had a score of 16 (*moderate depression*). Improvement in his depression-related symptoms was noted. Though Mr. Lewis acknowledged the improvement, he still expressed distress over his perceived inadequacies as a parent and problems with his daughter. The therapist asked Mr. Lewis how he thought people learned to be good parents. He felt that women somehow knew this intuitively but remembered that when his first child was a baby his wife frequently consulted her mother about how to handle problems that came up. The therapist asked if there was someone he could turn to for suggestions on parenting. He could think of none. "What about your own mother?" Mr. Lewis was puzzled because his mother was quite old but said that he would think about it. Returning again to the question of how care responsibilities were divided between himself and his daughter, Mr. Lewis said that he had told his daughter that he was frustrated having to care for the baby every day. An analysis of communication with his daughter revealed, however, that he always expressed his concerns in the midst of an argument. After an argument, to "have peace" he would drop the subject for fear it would lead to another argument. The therapist encouraged Mr. Lewis to think of other ways to discuss his concerns with his daughter. "Like what?" The therapist reviewed basic communication strategies such as discussing concerns outside of arguments, using *I* statements (vs. blaming *you* statements directed toward his daughter), thinking of a workable child-care plan that took account of his own needs as well as his daughter's, and containing angry affect in the context of a discussion. Mr. Lewis admitted that he was not very good at handling people but said it might be worth a try.

Session 9. Mr. Lewis seemed less depressed. He said that he asked his mother for ideas about how to handle a number of parenting problems he had with his grandchild. Much to his surprise, his mother was delighted that he sought her counsel and, in fact, offered a number of helpful suggestions about feeding, diapering, putting the baby to bed, and soothing his grandson when he was upset. The therapist asked if he had given any thought to how he might raise issues of concern with his daughter. He said he hadn't. The therapist encouraged further discussion of communication issues with his daughter and briefly role-played with Mr. Lewis a possible conversation. It was difficult for him as he quickly made blaming statements toward his daughter in the role play. The therapist gently pointed this out.

Session 10. Mr. Lewis said it had been a bad week with his daughter. They had had another argument over division of child-care responsibilities and he again apologized to her afterward even though he felt his daughter was wrong. The therapist helped Mr. Lewis to articulate what he felt was a fair division of responsibilities. He said that he was willing to take care of his grandson during the day when his daughter worked but felt that she should care for the baby in the evening and on the weekends. "Of course, I know there are times when she might want to see her friends in the evening. She needs friends but so do I. It would be okay if she did that sometimes but not every night." The therapist role-played a conversation with his daughter and Mr. Lewis showed some improvement in his communication skills. He noted at the end of the session that because of his mother's advice he felt he was handling things better with his grandson and that he felt less frustration about this. In fact, he had called his mother several times during the week asking for her advice. Even his daughter commented that he seemed to be doing better in caring for the baby.

Session 11. Mr. Lewis expressed continued frustration with the division of child-care responsibilities. He had planned to spend the weekend at his sister's weekend home but at the last minute his daughter told him that she needed his help caring for the baby because she wanted to work on Saturday to make some extra money. He said he had looked forward to a weekend away but felt he couldn't say anything because he had encouraged his daughter to save some money. "I said okay but I was mad at her all weekend." The therapist and Mr. Lewis discussed ways in which he might have communicated concerns to his daughter so that he could have gone away. He felt he was in a bind because he had complained to his daughter that she spent too much money and that if he didn't stay home she would "throw this in my face." Asked whether his daughter would in fact save the extra money, he said he hoped she would. It became apparent that Mr. Lewis and his daughter had never negotiated finances with each other and Mr. Lewis paid most bills. He said he was willing to do that "for a while." Asked how his daughter spent her money, he said he wasn't sure. Mr. Lewis said that he felt he needed to talk with his daughter about the division of responsibilities and during the remainder of the session the conversation was role-played.

Session 12. It had been a difficult week for Mr. Lewis because his grandson had another ear infection and needed to see the doctor again. The baby had problems sleeping several nights and Mr. Lewis didn't get much sleep. Nonetheless, he felt he was able to handle things better than he had and again called his mother for advice. He had spoken with his daughter about child-care arrangements and felt that things went "okay." "I said, 'Carrie, we need to talk. Is this a good time?' She said it was and I told her, 'Look, you know I love the baby and I love you. It's hard for me to take care of him during the day and then in the evenings and weekends.' My daughter shot back that she usually took care of him in the evenings and weekends. I tried to be calm. I told her, 'I know you usually do and I know it's hard for you working all day and then coming home to care for the baby. I need my time too and I want us to work something out.'" Eventually Mr. Lewis and his daughter found common ground in acknowledging how hard things had been for both of them in transitioning into parenting responsibilities. They both agreed that they each needed time away from the baby. He returned to Carrie's early suggestion that the baby could be placed in child care during the day. His daughter said that she hadn't realized how expensive it would be when she first raised the possibility and because of this did not raise the issue again with her father. "So we talked about how much it might cost and, she was right, it is expensive. Then I suggested to her that if she would pay half I would pay half. This way I could see my friends during the day and would be more willing to do babysitting on some evenings and weekends. Carrie said she'd think about it." Overall, Mr. Lewis felt that things were moving in the right direction. "But now let's see what Carrie does," he added.

Session 13. Carrie had set up an appointment to visit the child-care center. Tensions with her had eased. Mr. Lewis also took his grandson to spend part of a day with his mother. His mother had seen little of the baby because she had multiple medical problems and was generally homebound. The visit went especially well and Mr. Lewis thanked his mother for her guidance. "You're the last one I ever thought would change a diaper, Cal!" his mother remarked.

Termination

Session 14. The therapist reminded Mr. Lewis of the coming end of the therapy. He felt that the time had gone quickly, that in some ways "it seems like we just got started." When asked by the therapist about his feelings about ending, Mr. Lewis said that this wasn't a problem. The therapist said that some people found ending therapy upsetting but he denied this was the case for him. The therapist said that they would discuss the issue again in the remaining two sessions. Carrie had spoken with her father and they decided to enroll the baby in child care the following week. Mr. Lewis admitted that he had "second thoughts" about agreeing to pay for half the day care as he was on a limited income, but he felt it would be worth it. There was discussion with Carrie about arrangements for delivery and retrieval of the baby from day care.

Session 15. In this penultimate session, Mr. Lewis reported that he began to take his grandson to child care. Much to his surprise two other older adults were delivering children to the center. The therapist asked Mr. Lewis whether he had any thoughts about the fact there would be only one more planned session. He said that, in fact, he was nervous about ending and wondered whether sessions might continue for a while. The therapist explored his concerns and found that Mr. Lewis was feeling anxious about the end of the therapy and wondered whether he was becoming depressed. The therapist clarified that this did not appear to be the case but that apprehension about ending was normal. The therapist told Mr. Lewis that he was impressed with the progress that he had made in therapy and that he felt optimistic about Mr. Lewis's future. It also appeared that Mr. Lewis's depressive symptoms had improved considerably and would be formally evaluated in the final session.

Session 16. The therapist conducted the HRSD. "Mr. Lewis, your score is now 6 on this depression scale. It was 22 when you started. You have very few depressive symptoms now and are no longer in a major depression." Mr. Lewis expressed relief about this news and also gratitude toward the therapist. "I think you should be most grateful to yourself. You came into therapy feeling quite depressed and overwhelmed by the new responsibilities for care of your grandson. Your new parenting role led to difficulties with your daughter, which made things all the more difficult. You thought through the problems you faced, got help from your mother in figuring out ways to deal with the many issues that come up when caring for a baby, and followed through on her suggestions. You also thought long and hard about how to talk with your daughter about a better child-care arrangement. You've done a lot of work and your progress shows." Mr. Lewis said he acknowledged that things were going much better but still wanted to continue to see the therapist. They agreed to see each other in maintenance therapy. Following the end of therapy Mr. Lewis saw the therapist every other week for 2 months, then monthly for 6 more months at which time he terminated psychotherapy.

Case Commentary

A critical goal for Mr. Lewis was acquiring needed skills to master his role as parent to his grandson. With increased mastery over the role he could see his new role in a more positive light and, in fact, take more satisfaction in contact with his daughter and grandson. It is interesting that Mr. Lewis learned important parenting skills from his mother. With a renegotiation of child-care arrangements with his daughter, he was able to reclaim some of the social and recreational activities associated with his "old role"—that is, his role as a retired man with few daily responsibilities. Issues related to the secondary problem area, interpersonal role disputes, were intertwined with his role transition into parenting. He and his daughter had not clearly delineated the parameters of their coparenting of the baby. Failure to do so resulted in confusion of expectations, which was fertile ground for the development of a dispute. In some ways, the issues reflect some of those evident in younger couples who must negotiate child-care responsibilities with each other. Among IPT's techniques, exploration, clarification, and communication analysis were most helpful in implementing strategies outlined for role transitions and interpersonal role disputes.

CONCLUDING COMMENTARY

As noted earlier, we find role acquisition rather than role loss (such as retirement) to be the most common treatment issue in this IPT problem area. Of course, acquisition of a new role usually results in loss of or change in old roles. Mrs. Barton's case illustrates common problems for individuals transitioning into the role of dementia caregiver. Many family members initially find it hard to accept that a close relative has dementia. Older adults know that they and older family members are at increasing risk for dementia as they age and many fear that it will happen. If dementia does enter their lives, acceptance of that reality is a gradual process. Feelings of fear and grief are normal—feelings that need to be acknowledged as part of the process of acceptance. Managing home health aides can be stressful, especially for individuals who have had no prior experience in managing employees. Some older people take on primary child-care responsibilities in later life, a phenomenon that is more common in African American communities than in other racial or ethnic communities (Pruchno, 1999). In a similar way, acquisition of a parenting role in later life usually confronts the older person with responsibilities that were not anticipated, perhaps disappointment with life choices that an adult child has made that require the client's parenting assistance, and the need to give up aspects of the current pattern of living. As Mr. Lewis's case illustrates, for those with limited parenting experience, the new role also requires acquisition of new skills as well as negotiation of responsibilities with an adult child.

9

INTERPERSONAL DEFICITS

A large research literature has convincingly documented that social relationships have a positive effect on physical health, mental health, and risk for mortality (George, 2004). As discussed in chapter 2, interpersonally relevant events are tied to increased risk of depression in older adults (George, 1994; Hinrichsen & Emery, 2005). As mentioned in chapter 1 (this volume), most older adults have reasonably well-developed social ties. A minority of older adults, however, have poorly developed social relationships that have been evident throughout their lives or become evident in late life. The origins of poor social ties are many, including age-related loss of social relationships, psychiatric conditions such as schizoid personality disorder and other personality disorders, and interpersonal deficits. The focus of this interpersonal psychotherapy (IPT) problem area is individuals with interpersonal deficits. These individuals have difficulty in initiating and sustaining relationships despite a desire to have them. They usually feel isolated, lonely, and depressed as a result.

We see few older adults for whom the primary problem is interpersonal deficits. Most older adults seek mental health treatment at the behest of family or friends. Often lacking substantive relationships, individuals with interpersonal deficits are therefore less likely to access treatment in outpatient mental health settings. As a community social service outreach worker early in his career, Hinrichsen would sometimes meet individuals with interpersonal deficits. When depression was evident, they might accept referral

153

for mental health services but required considerable encouragement and support to do so. Multiple home visits by mental health workers were often needed to establish an initial relationship with the client who could then transition into clinic-based treatment. Treatment would then focus on improvement of depression and development of better social ties. Some colleagues who work in Department of Veterans Affairs facilities informally tell us that individuals with interpersonal deficits are sometimes referred by primary care medical care providers because absence of social ties impedes compliance with medical regimens or contributes to mental health problems including depression. Nursing home psychologists also report that lifelong social isolates are part of the mix of residents. Relocation to a nursing home for persons with interpersonal deficits can be especially challenging as they confront the complex world of the nursing home that includes ongoing interaction with staff and other residents. They lack the social skills needed to contend with these interpersonal demands and at the same time are experiencing one or more medical problems that prompted the nursing home placement.

In outpatient clinical practice, a life crisis such as the loss of a critical relationship and associated depression may motivate the individual to seek services. The loss of a family member or friend—whether from death, relocation, or disability—on whom the individual exclusively relied may leave the individual quite alone and lacking the interpersonal resources to initiate a new relationship. Some unmarried or divorced older persons who lived with aging parents throughout most of their lives and without other ties may confront an interpersonal developmental crisis as they enter the later years (Rubinstein, 1987; Rubinstein, Alexander, Goodman, & Luborsky, 1991). Although they may be experiencing feelings of grief, the critical issue is their subjective perception that "I have no one." Depression may follow. Some men, particularly those without children or who have estranged relationships with their children and who have exclusively relied on their wives to facilitate social ties, may find themselves socially isolated after the death of their wife, and lacking the knowledge or skills to make social connections.

Acute IPT treatment for interpersonal deficits can be useful to begin establishing social connections with a concurrent reduction in depressive symptoms. Our experience and that of others (Weissman, Markowitz, & Klerman, 2000) suggests that continued psychotherapeutic work is needed following acute treatment. Especially for those with lifelong interpersonal deficits, ongoing support from the therapist helps to further build social relations that reduce the likelihood of recurrence of another episode of depression.

GOALS AND STRATEGIES IN THE IPT TREATMENT OF INTERPERSONAL DEFICITS

The goals of IPT in this problem area are to reduce social isolation and encourage the formation of new relationships (see Exhibit 9.1). Social isola-

EXHIBIT 9.1
Outline of Interpersonal Psychotherapy for Major Depression

D. Interpersonal Deficits
  1. Goals
     a. Reduce the patient's social isolation.
     b. Encourage formation of new relationships.
  2. Strategies
     a. Review depressive symptoms.
     b. Relate depressive symptoms to problems of social isolation or unfulfill-ment.
     c. Review past significant relationships including their negative and positive aspects.
     d. Explore repetitive patterns in relationships.
     e. Discuss patient's positive and negative feelings about therapist and seek parallels in other relationships.

Note. From Comprehensive Guide to Interpersonal Psychotherapy (p. 24), by M. M. Weissman, J. C. Markowitz, and G. L. Klerman, 2000, New York: Basic Books. Copyright 2000 by Basic Books. Reprinted with permission.

tion may be reduced by increasing opportunities for the client to simply be in the presence of other individuals. Initially opportunities may be as basic as being around other people (vs. staying alone at home) even if the client does not talk with other individuals. Being in the presence of other people may be beneficial to mood and begin to build some initial confidence in dealing with people. For example, a client might be encouraged to attend a lecture, go to a movie, have a meal at a senior center, spend time in the common area of a nursing home, attend religious services, or go to a shopping center. Social involvements that require more interpersonal interaction include part-time employment or a volunteer job. Formation of new relationships is a longer term project in which the therapist works with the client to build basic skills for interacting with other people and sustaining nascent relation-ships. The therapist uses a great deal of role-playing and communication analysis techniques. The therapist often gives direct feedback to the client about his or her interactional style with the therapist.

Strategies 2a and 2b: Review depressive symptoms. Relate depressive symptoms to problems of social isolation or unfulfillment. As with all of the problem areas, depressive symptoms are reviewed in the initial sessions and reviewed again throughout therapy. The connection between depressive symptoms and problems in social engagement is made explicit in the initial sessions and reiterated during the middle sessions. It is useful for the client to understand that depression itself will make it more difficult to function socially. With improvement in depressive symptoms, the client should find it easier to engage socially.

Strategy 2c: Review past significant relationships including their negative and positive aspects. Although the interpersonal inventory is conducted in the initial sessions, the therapist facilitates a more detailed discussion of relationships in the middle sessions. Because the client has no or few current relationships, an understanding of past relationships assumes greater importance than it does in other IPT problem areas. By discussing past relationships, both the therapist and client are able to gain a deeper understanding of what the client has done in the past that promotes better or worse interpersonal functioning. For example, a client might demonstrate adequate skill in establishing relationships but have problems in sustaining them. Or perhaps, despite a history of many failed relationships, one relationship has endured for several years. Interpersonal behavior evident in that relationship may be emulated to help develop future relationships. More likely, the client will recount negative aspects of relationships. The therapist should focus on specific difficulties that emerged in past significant relationships, as this information will help to clarify the client's current interpersonal skills deficits.

Strategy 2d: Explore repetitive patterns in relationships. With information gleaned from Strategy 2c, the therapist will be in a better position to identify repetitive interpersonal problems. For the therapist, this understanding provides a framework for discerning where the client has had problems in initiating or sustaining relationships. Some themes that may emerge include inability to successfully negotiate differences; attribution of negative intentions to another person when there is no good evidence for it; avoidance of relationships because of a conviction that one is unlikable, unattractive, and uninteresting; and a failure to evidence basic social skills such as showing interest in the other person, taking the other person's perspective, or, conversely, inability to assert one's own interests or preferences.

Strategy 2e: Discuss patient's positive and negative feelings about therapist and seek parallels in other relationships. As mentioned earlier, the relationship with the therapist assumes greater importance than it does in other problem areas. IPT does not use interpretations of transferential behavior on the part of the client toward the therapist as a therapeutic intervention. In this problem area, however, clarification and problem-solving of therapist–client issues can facilitate the development of interpersonal skills that the client can use in daily life. It is likely that the interpersonal theme or themes from past relationships will be replayed with the therapist. By drawing parallels between issues that emerge with the therapist and in other relationships, the client can be mindful of these interpersonal problems and work with the therapist to develop skills to improve them. The therapist can also give direct feedback to the client about interpersonal behavior (i.e., "you don't make much eye contact when you speak," "despite your conviction you are boring, you actually speak in an animated and interesting way to me," "you may be unaware of it, but there is often an angry tone to your voice").

Establishment of the therapeutic relationship with those who have interpersonal deficits may be more difficult than with clients who have other problems, yet, once established, the relationship can be used to assist the client to improve even long-standing social deficits. As persons with interpersonal deficits may be shunned or avoided by others, the therapist may be one of the few people in the client's entire life who has given them encouragement and honest feedback on how they handle interpersonal relations. Identification of specific problems and interpersonal strategies to address them can reduce self-blame, engender hopefulness, and reduce depression. As noted, continuation of psychotherapy beyond the acute phase is usually indicated to further build skills and provide encouragement, but this should not be decided until the termination phase of treatment. As mentioned earlier, the time pressure of brief treatment can motivate the client to change.

CONTINUATION OF THE CASE OF RACHEL GREENBERG

Discussion of the initial session of this case can be found in chapter 5 (this volume). To recap: Ms. Greenberg is a 62-year-old, never-married woman with scoliosis who experienced the onset of depressive symptoms after the death of her mother. She was diagnosed with major depression, single episode, severe with a Hamilton Rating Scale for Depression (HRSD) score of 27. Although she was experiencing feelings of grief related to her mother's death, her chief concern was her social isolation. She felt that connections were increasingly important as she reckoned with the reality that she was entering later adulthood.

Intermediate Sessions

Session 4. As the session began, the therapist inquired about Ms. Greenberg's mood. She said that she was feeling more depressed and did not know why. To get more details, the therapist asked what had happened during the week. She reported that she had done little. The therapist then asked what she had done on each day of the past week. She had done some shopping and had visited her brother briefly but little more than that. The therapist pointed out that her depressive illness made it more difficult for her to function but that lack of activities and contact with others also contributed to the depression. Ms. Greenberg said that she thought of looking for a job and had glanced through the help-wanted section of the newspaper. She had worked in a clerical capacity for a governmental agency for most of her life but took early retirement when her mother became ill. Her pension was modest and she needed money to supplement it. The therapist noted that employment would put her into contact with others and help to reduce social isolation. Ms. Greenberg acknowledged this but said that she had been disappointed with people she knew from the job from which she retired. At this point the therapist felt it would be useful to review her history of social relations at work. At first Ms. Greenberg spoke vaguely and globally about disappointments with others, with the predominant theme that others did not like her or take her seriously. The therapist tried to focus on specific relationships about which she had discontent. "When I first worked for the agency, I really liked my supervisor Joan. She always looked out for me and said that I did good work. After a while she started avoiding me." Asked why that might be, Mrs. Greenberg said she did not know; perhaps it was because of her appearance. When asked what aspect of her appearance might have bothered her former supervisor, she looked annoyed. "Why, my back, of course!" The therapist told Ms. Greenberg that he couldn't be certain what part of her appearance she was referring to. This was the reason he needed to ask her directly. "From what you've said before, having scoliosis has been something that has bothered you throughout your life. I think it would be helpful to talk about that." "What good would that do?" "Well, it seems that you feel that some people don't like you because of the scoliosis. Because you're interested in making connections with others and you feel this gets in the way, it might help to discuss it." Ms. Greenberg said "Maybe," and changed the topic. She ended the session complaining about her sister-in-law who, she reminded the therapist, had once called her "pathetic." On her visit to her brother's home, she said her sister-in-law criticized her for wanting to renovate her kitchen. "What business is it of hers?" remarked Ms. Greenberg but then said she wondered whether she really needed to redo the kitchen.

Session 5. Ms. Greenberg started the next session recounting a litany of complaints about her sister-in-law. There had been another incident in which her sister-in-law said that she was foolish to waste money on renovating her kitchen. It appeared that Ms. Greenberg's mood worsened following these interactions. The therapist noted this connection. The therapist continued the discussion of Ms. Greenberg's past work relationships. It appeared that, on the whole, she was a competent and reliable worker. At first she had congenial relations with coworkers but, at some point, for reasons unknown to her, relationships would become more distant. Then she would become hurt and angry and further distance herself from coworkers. The therapist asked whether she felt that coworkers had rejected her because of her appearance as she felt that her supervisor Joan had. "Probably." "I'm curious, Ms. Greenberg. If they were rejecting you because of your appearance, why were they friendly with you to begin with?" "They were probably feeling sorry for me and then got tired of me. I'm pretty boring. Sometimes I go to family gatherings and after a while the person I'm talking to just drifts off to talk to another person." "And why would that be?" asked the therapist. "Because I'm boring. I told you that!" said Ms. Greenberg with annoyance. "I'm sure that there are times when other people may not be interested in what you are saying. There are a lot of reasons why a person may seem to lose interest in a conversation. What strikes me is that you usually assume it's because of you. I'm not totally convinced of that. I think it would be helpful to talk more about your interactions with other people during our work together."

Session 6. Ms. Greenberg reported feeling less depressed. Asked what had happened in the prior week, she said that she answered an ad in the newspaper and had a job interview. She admitted that she was feeling nervous about going for a job interview. When the therapist said that they could role-play the job interview, she was very interested. She expressed fear that she would freeze up, sound boring, or appear incompetent. The therapist reviewed with her what she knew about the job and what she would like to learn about the job including hours, responsibilities, and salary. The therapist role-played the job interviewer. He offered feedback on what she said and suggestions on how to phrase questions. On the whole she conducted herself fairly well in the role play. The therapist noted that improvement in depressive symptoms seemed tied to actions she had taken to secure a job. She acknowledged this but expressed fears that she might not get the job.

Session 7. Ms. Greenberg announced that she had secured part-time employment. She said that she was very pleased with this but was now nervous about how well she would perform. After discussion of ways to manage her anxiety when starting the job, Mrs. Greenberg remarked, "This must be a very hard job. You have to listen to everybody's problems. I'll bet sometimes you don't want to come to work." The therapist encouraged her to discuss further the thoughts she was having about him. At first, she was reluctant but then alluded to how listening to people's problems was probably boring. "Do you think I'm bored with you?" asked the therapist. "Why wouldn't you be?" Ms. Greenberg noted that in the previous session the therapist had yawned, which convinced her that he was bored with her. At this point the therapist decided to give direct feedback to Ms. Greenberg. "Ms. Greenberg, I don't, in fact, find you boring. I was likely yawning last week because it was late in the afternoon when I sometimes feel a little sleepy. Despite what you think about yourself, I find that you've discussed relevant issues during our sessions and am impressed with the fact that you have secured a job. I think you're moving in the right direction." She said that what the therapist said was "very nice" but that he likely said it because "you feel sorry for me." "I don't feel sorry for you. I have concern about you and want to work with you so that you are less depressed and have better connections. But I do not feel sorry for you."

Session 8. In this mid-therapy session, the therapist conducted the HRSD, on which she had a score of 17 (*moderate depression*)—a reduction of 10 points from the beginning of therapy. Her sleep and appetite as well as her functioning had significantly improved. The therapist noted the improvement and said that it could likely be attributed to her efforts to gain employment, clarifying and problem-solving issues in therapy, and the effects of the antidepressant medication. The therapist reviewed the past week's events with Ms. Greenberg. Work seemed to be going reasonably well despite anxiety about her performance. Coworkers "seemed nice" but she was disappointed that they had not invited her out to lunch. With encouragement, Ms. Greenberg acknowledged she could take the initiative of asking a coworker out to lunch but was afraid of rebuff. The therapist encouraged Ms. Greenberg to talk more about her history of relationships with others. She said that she had pleasant recollections of her childhood and her relationship with other children. She attended private schools through the seventh grade. Then her parents had financial difficulties and she transferred to a public school. "At that point my whole life changed. Starting from the first day at school kids began to make fun of me. They laughed at my back, called me names. I tried to fight back but that only made things worse." During high school she had no close relationships, did not take part in extracurricular activities, and spent all of her free time with family. The therapist empathized with how painful those years must have been for her and how increasingly mental health care professionals and school official have understood the damaging impact of bullying on young people. Ms. Greenberg said that she had read in the paper about high school children who had been bullied and then shot their classmates. "I would never have done that but I understand why they did it." The therapist helped Ms. Greenberg clarify and understand feelings of anger she felt about her treatment during her adolescence.

Session 9. Ms. Greenberg said she continued to feel better and that despite her fears, work still seemed to be going fairly well. In fact, a coworker had invited her out to lunch. The therapist encouraged her to continue discussing her history of social relationships. In young adulthood, she socialized primarily with her parents and their relatives. "I liked the older people because they were the most understanding." She had established one or two friendships from work which had, in fact, endured for several years. The friendships seemed to have ended when a problem emerged in the relationship. Instead of talking about the problem, Ms. Greenberg withdrew. "They probably never liked me anyway." The therapist challenged this statement. "Why would they have been friends with you for so many years if they did not like you to begin with?" Ms. Greenberg said she knew this statement "didn't make sense" and asked the therapist how he would explain her social problems. "Here's what I think," began the therapist. "From what you've said you had good relations with your peers before you changed schools. It sounds like you were scapegoated by your peers because you were new to the school and you had scoliosis, and for other reasons that neither of us could know. You withdrew to your family, depriving yourself of the opportunity to develop the skills that most younger people do in interactions with peers. You left high school with the conviction that you were unattractive and boring. As an adult, you assumed that other people would treat you as you were treated in high school. You therefore avoided relations with people outside of your family. On the basis of your experiences from school days, you have a conviction that it's only a matter of time before you will be rejected. The same thing happened between us. Remember when you thought you were boring me?" Ms. Greenberg said that this formulation made sense to her. "But what do I do about it?" "We will continue to work together so that you can learn how to better manage your relationships with others—including your own anxieties—so that you have better connections with people. Look at what you've done already—you got a job and are with people most days of the week. And, you're feeling better."

Session 10. Ms. Greenberg said that she had had lunch again with the coworker who invited her out. "Things didn't go so well this time. I think she found me boring." When the specifics of the luncheon engagement were reviewed, it became apparent that Ms. Greenberg was less talkative and engaged than she had been at the prior lunch date with her coworker. She said that she did not know what to say and feared that if she said something, her coworker would find her uninteresting. The therapist reviewed assumptions about herself that she brought into relationships and how these likely created anxiety that, in turn, made her "less natural" in her dealings with others. Therapist and client reviewed topics that she could bring up in a conversation to "keep it going": politics, current events, things she had seen on television, events at work, books she had read.

Session 11. Ms. Greenberg said she had been a bit more depressed in the prior week despite the fact that she had lunch again with the coworker and that things went more smoothly and she felt more comfortable. "I hate my sister-in-law." There had been another incident in which her sister-in-law treated her disrespectfully. "I went ahead and remodeled the kitchen. She insisted on seeing it and when she did, she said she didn't like it." It appeared from what Ms. Greenberg had said that indeed her sister-in-law was a difficult person. The therapist engaged the client in a discussion of how to be assertive. She really did not want her sister-in-law to come to her home, but she did not know how to say no. Ways in which she could have done this politely and firmly were discussed, and Ms. Greenberg found the discussion helpful. She said that whenever she visited her brother, her sister-in-law would sometime make a critical statement about Ms. Greenberg. She said she loved her brother dearly but felt his wife got in the way of their relationship. The therapist encouraged her to think of ways in which she could spend time alone with her brother. Eventually she decided that she would ask her brother to have dinner with her once a month. Ms. Greenberg said that she was interested in meeting some people in addition to those from work. Different options for doing this were discussed. With each option, she expressed apprehension that she did not know how to start a conversation with someone she did not know and fears of "freezing up" and "sounding boring." It appeared that one route to increased social contact would be one in which there was some common denominator among the participants. Ms. Greenberg said she would think about what might be another viable social option.

Session 12. Ms. Greenberg began the session by saying that she had been thinking about the fact that the psychotherapy was for only 16 weeks. She expressed apprehension about what would happen at the end of the therapy. "What will I do without you?" Ms. Greenberg said that she had grown to rely on the therapist for advice and wondered how she would handle things on her own. The therapist noted that the last 3 weeks of therapy time would be dedicated to discuss these very issues. He pointed out that she had done well during the course of the therapy: Her depressive symptoms continued to decrease and she had made concrete efforts to reduce social isolation. Nonetheless, he said he understood Ms. Greenberg's apprehension, that other clients felt apprehension about ending therapy, and that her progress at the end of therapy would be assessed, and, at that point, options would be explored regarding any additional assistance she might need or want. She said that she was feeling a bit more depressed during the past week thinking about this issue. Work generally went well but she thought that her boss was "hinting" to her that her work was subpar. "I think she feels sorry for me so she won't tell me directly." Ms. Greenberg did, in fact, have some difficulties correctly taking messages from phone calls. Her eyesight was getting poorer because of cataracts and she thought this contributed to some work problems. After discussion, the therapist asked if Ms. Greenberg felt comfortable directly asking her supervisor for feedback on her work. They role-played this conversation. On leaving the session Ms. Greenberg said that she had asked her brother to have dinner and he accepted. She hadn't thought about a way to find another avenue for socialization other than work.

Session 13. Ms. Greenberg reported that she had had a conversation with her boss about her performance. Indeed her boss did have concerns that phone messages had not been legibly or accurately written. Ms. Greenberg explained the problem with her failing vision and the supervisor assured her that she could take time off when needed to have cataract surgery. She was relieved by the conversation but in some ways it confirmed her suspicion that others were harboring negative thoughts about her. "And then all of a sudden things end." The therapist said that indeed sometimes people do have concerns that they don't convey. However, Ms. Greenberg had a propensity to assume—without much information—that most people thought poorly of her. In this case she correctly perceived concerns that her boss had about her performance—concerns that she herself also had. Instead of avoiding the supervisor and becoming increasingly anxious about the issue, she directly asked for feedback, which led to a productive conversation. She had a generally enjoyable dinner with her brother in the prior week. "He dropped a bomb, however. He said that he was beginning to think about retiring and when he did he would probably move to his summer home in another state. He said that I could move with him and his wife. But I couldn't stand living with that woman." Even though her brother's departure was likely several years away, it raised anxiety about "who will take care of me when I'm old." The therapist noted that though her brother's retirement was well into the future, it was of obvious concern to her now. If her brother did move, different options were reviewed, including remaining where she currently lived and visiting him often, moving to an assisted living residence when she became much older, or moving into a separate residence near his out-of-state home.

Termination

Session 14. Ms. Greenberg said that in the prior week she had thought about another way to meet people. She learned about a monthly book club at her local library. She enjoyed reading and thought the book club would be a more comfortable way to meet other people. The therapist congratulated her on finding a vehicle for socializing with people in which all had a common topic of interest—the book that was being read that month. She expressed concern that other members might find her comments uninteresting. The therapist pointed out that this was an ongoing concern of hers. During the course of therapy she, in fact, had mentioned some books she had been reading and the therapist thought that she made rather astute comments. Transitioning into a discussion of termination, the therapist noted the fact that two sessions remained. He said he knew that Ms. Greenberg had thoughts and feelings about the end of the treatment. "Why is this only 16 weeks?" she asked. "Do you limit it to 16 weeks with all of your patients?" The therapist noted that the length of treatment depended on the kind of therapy the therapist was using and the kind of difficulties a client was experiencing. Sensing that Ms. Greenberg was indirectly raising an issue, the therapist asked, "Do you think that this therapy is 16 weeks for other reasons?" She paused and said, "Well, I did wonder whether you were ending things because I was boring. I know that's what I always wonder and maybe that's not true. But it did cross my mind." The therapist said that he wasn't surprised that this thought came to her mind because she often wondered about this in relationships. He noted that the time frame for treatment had been established from the outset and was based on research studies that found that 16 weeks was useful for most people in significantly reducing depressive symptoms and in improving their ability to deal with life problems. She expressed apprehension about ending and wondered how she could handle things by herself. Improvement in depressive symptoms, acquisition of a job, a slowly developing relationship with a coworker, and plans to attend the library book club were noted as accomplishments by the therapist. She acknowledged these accomplishments but reiterated apprehension about the end of therapy. The therapist finished the session by inquiring about depressive symptoms which Ms. Greenberg felt had increased in the prior week as a result of worries about ending therapy.

Session 15. The therapist inquired about symptoms. Ms. Greenberg said she was feeling more nervous and "upset" and wondered whether she was getting depressed again. After review of symptoms, she did not, in fact, evidence increased depressive symptoms—in fact, they were much decreased relative to entry into therapy. "Ms. Greenberg, what you call an increase in depression is actually understandable apprehension about ending therapy. This sometimes happens. I think you've done well and expect that you will continue to do better." "I know I'm doing better," she replied, "but it's just that . . . well, I lost my mother and now I'm losing you." The therapist was not surprised that Ms. Greenberg had begun to look to the therapist in a way that had parallels with her relationship with her mother. She would likely benefit from additional treatment but the therapist was mindful of the possibility that she might overly rely on the therapeutic relationship in a way that would reduce the incentive to establish connections with others. The therapist acknowledged her feelings of attachment to him but noted that the therapeutic relationship was different from a friendship. Ms. Greenberg said that she understood that but felt that she needed additional help from the therapist despite the improvement she had made. The therapist said that in the final session they would review treatment options. At the end of the session she noted that she had attended the library book club and although she said little during the meeting the other participants seemed "nice."

Session 16. The therapist began with administration of the HRSD, on which she had a score of 7, which is in the nondepressed range. Ms. Greenberg said that she was indeed much less depressed and felt that she had made progress in therapy. The therapist noted that depressive symptoms had significantly diminished and that she no longer met criteria for a major depression. The therapist reviewed the essentials of her course in treatment: onset of a major depressive illness following feelings of social isolation; the goals of treatment including reduction of depressive symptoms and enhancement of social functioning; her active efforts within therapy (as well as taking prescribed antidepressant medication) to improve these problems; and significant improvement in depressive symptoms. "You've helped me so much." "You've helped yourself so much," replied the therapist. "Now what?" asked Ms. Greenberg. "What do you want?" "I would like to continue to see you," she replied. The therapist reiterated his concerns about the therapeutic relationship becoming a substitute for other relationships and said that if therapy were to continue it was important to have clear goals for further enhancement of her social functioning. Reasonable goals of sustained improvement in depressive symptoms and further enlargement of social relationships were established with Ms. Greenberg.

Post–Acute Phase Treatment

The therapist and Ms. Greenberg continued to meet weekly for another 16 weeks. Therapy built on gains she had made during acute treatment. Issues in a developing relationship with a coworker were clarified and IPT techniques of communication analysis and role play were often used. Prior to attendance at book club meetings, Ms. Greenberg would review what she wanted to say about the book and strategies for engaging with other members of the book club after the meeting. She planned a 3-day tour of Washington, DC, for older adults with a travel agency. Therapist and client discussed in detail social circumstances that she would encounter with other members of the tour and role-played a number of scenarios. During the tour she developed a budding relationship with another older woman which she then nourished by taking other tours with the woman. At the end of the second 16 weeks of IPT, Ms. Greenberg agreed to participate in a weekly group psychotherapy for older adults and individual sessions were reduced to monthly visits. After 6 months of monthly visits, individual IPT was ended although Ms. Greenberg continued in group psychotherapy.

Case Commentary

Consistent with the goals of IPT treatment of interpersonal deficits, Ms. Greenberg reduced social isolation by taking a job and joining the book club. By the end of acute treatment, she had the beginnings of a relationship with a coworker. In accordance with IPT strategies, her depressive symptoms were reviewed on an ongoing basis and the connection between depression and social isolation was noted. A review of negative and positive aspects of past relationships was especially fruitful in gaining an understanding of repetitive patterns in her relationships. She expected that others would think negatively of her (i.e., boring, unattractive) and that if they engaged with her it would be out of pity. For relationships that endured for some period, she anticipated the end of them when others "finally" discovered or "tired" of her negative attributes. When inevitable relationship issues did arise, she misattributed problems and she did not possess the skills to successfully negotiate differences. Anxiety about these issues further contributed to her social awkwardness. The onset of major depression also impeded her ability to initiate or sustain social relationships. Some of these issues arose, not unexpectedly, in the context of the therapeutic relationship and were addressed.

Ms. Greenberg developed attachment to the therapist and expressed the desire to continue in therapy. On the basis of the experience of other IPT therapists in treating interpersonal deficits (Weissman et al., 2000) and the documented usefulness of IPT maintenance therapies in reducing relapse and recurrence of major depression, continuing the treatment was clinically indicated. The problem that the therapist faced was how to continue therapy in a manner that promoted enhancement of Ms. Greenberg's social competence versus increasing reliance on the therapist for support and encouragement that might replicate the relationship with her mother. The therapist explicitly discussed this concern and maintained sharp focus on the further development of social skills during the second 16 weeks of treatment. Eventual transition into group psychotherapy provided ongoing opportunities for Ms. Greenberg to get feedback from other group members about her interpersonal behavior. The group also provided a place where she could get support and encouragement from age peers.

CASE EXAMPLE: BOB HOLDEN

Mr. Holden was a 78-year-old, divorced retired plumber who had been a resident of the nursing home for about 2 years. On evaluation, the therapist noted marked psychomotor retardation and found that he had major depression, moderate with an HRSD score of 17 (*moderate depression*). He likely had one more episodes of untreated major depression but it was difficult to document. The onset of the depression was 6 months earlier and appeared to have coincided with the end of visits from a friend, Charlie, who, because of physical infirmity, had moved out-of-state to live with an adult child. Mr. Holden had a history of colon cancer that necessitated use of a colostomy bag. In addition, he had cardiac problems and arthritis. In initial sessions, he acknowledged that there was a problem with the changing of his colostomy bag, which he attributed to poor nursing care. The aide who changed the bag often came late and because of that he did it himself. The therapist spoke with nursing staff who said they also thought he was depressed but he had refused antidepressant medication. "He's totally noncooperative," said a floor nurse sharply. However, further discussion with the nurse revealed that uncooperative behavior had emerged only in recent months and that previously he had been a withdrawn, unremarkable resident. In fact, Mr. Holden was referred by nursing staff to the psychologist who worked as a consultant in the nursing home where Mr. Holden resided because he insisted on changing his colostomy bag by himself, which often resulted in feces discharging onto the floor and into his bed. Nursing staff had repeatedly asked Mr. Holden to wait for them to change his bag but he did not. The essence of the referral was "make him stop this."

Conduct of the interpersonal inventory revealed marked paucity of relationships throughout his life. He described an unhappy childhood in which his father was physically abusive to his mother, his siblings, and himself. He had divorced early in his life and had no children. Although he desired to remarry he was not successful in finding another mate. He had two siblings but they had very little contact. A nephew became reluctantly involved in facilitating his move to the nursing home when his doctor called the family because he became alarmed over Mr. Holden's inability to care for himself at home. Mr. Holden had one friend, Charlie, whom he had met through work. He and Charlie went to the racetrack to bet on horses and sometimes went to a local tavern to watch sports on television.

Intermediate Sessions

Session 4. Although it had been discussed in the initial sessions, the therapist again reviewed her understanding of Mr. Holden's circumstances. She did this because in the initial sessions Mr. Holden only reluctantly acknowledged that he was depressed. "As we talked about, you have a major depression which developed after Charlie moved away. It seems to me that you've always had problems connecting with people and that Charlie's move away has been very hard for you. Being depressed makes it even harder to deal with his move and also cope with living in the nursing home." Mr. Holden nodded in agreement yet quickly changed the topic. "That damn nurse aide. She was late again to change the colostomy bag. I changed it myself and then she yelled at me because of the mess. I told her to get the hell out of my room." The therapist pressed for details and found that conflict over changing of the colostomy bag emerged only in recent months when there was a change in nursing aides. He characterized the new nursing aide as "lazy" yet acknowledged that the previous aide had been late at times in changing the bag. The therapist asked for additional details of their interactions, during the course of which Mr. Holden referred to the aide as "those people." "Which people are you referring to?" asked the therapist. "Blacks," he said. He acknowledged that he held negative views toward racial minorities and admitted that during one of his first disputes with the aide he used a racial slur. "And after that it seemed like she deliberately tried to be late." Mr. Holden said he regretted making the remark and understood why she wouldn't like him but still felt she should be on time. The therapist encouraged Mr. Holden to think of some ways in which difficulties with the aide might be improved during the upcoming week.

Session 5. Mr. Holden said he was feeling a little better in the past week. Referring to the therapist, he said it was "good to talk to somebody" and that he did indeed miss Charlie's visits. Charlie had, in fact, called him during the week, which made him feel better. The therapist asked if he had given thought to how to improve things with the aide. "I'll bet you want me to apologize to her." "Do you want to apologize?" asked the therapist. "No, she should apologize to me." Different options were discussed for handling the situation. Finally a decision was made to have a joint meeting with Mr. Holden, the aide, and the therapist the next week. The therapist and client discussed what Mr. Holden wanted to say to the aide and what he wanted to accomplish through the conversation. "To get her to come on time." "Okay, how can you accomplish that?" He acknowledged that it would be difficult to talk to the aide without getting upset but would try to hold his anger in check. He asked the therapist to help him during the conversation. The session ended with further discussion of past significant relationships in his life. He appeared to have had a particularly difficult relationship with his father whom he referred to as "that son of a bitch."

Session 6. Both Mr. Holden and the aide appeared nervous. The therapist began the meeting. "I understand both you and Mr. Holden have been concerned about when and how his colostomy bag has been changed." The aide detailed the problems she faced in cleaning up when Mr. Holden changed the bag himself, her own feelings of being overwhelmed by the many residents for whom she was responsible, and how she deserved "respect" from all residents. "Do you feel that Mr. Holden has acted disrespectfully toward you?" asked the therapist. The aide stared angrily at Mr. Holden and then a tear rolled down her face. She said he had called her a terrible name. Mr. Holden softened and he said, "I'm sorry that I said that to you." The aide composed herself. She said that she would make every effort to arrive on time to change his bag and that if she were running late she would drop by the room and tell him when she would likely come by. After the aide left Mr. Holden said that he had not intended to hurt the aide's feelings and that he, himself, knew what it was like to be treated disrespectfully. He gave a history of physical abuse as a child by his father, being called demeaning names and told "you won't amount to anything." He witnessed similar treatment directed toward his mother and siblings. "How do you think that affected you in your life?" Mr. Holden just shook his head. "I'm not very good with people."

Session 7. The therapist inquired about Mr. Holden's mood. He said he'd been feeling better, "less depressed as you would say." The aide had been on time most of the week. He expressed appreciation for the therapist's intervention. She pointed out that Mr. Holden had contained his anger in the meeting and acknowledged the aide's feelings. His efforts as much as the therapist's had improved his relationship with the aide. Returning to further discussion of past significant relationships, Mr. Holden said that things had gone well with his wife in the first year of their marriage. Much to his distress, however, he found himself increasingly losing his temper with his wife. "When I hit her, she left me." He had a series of brief, failed relationships with other women and "finally gave up trying." On holidays he would make an appearance at family gatherings but did not make enduring connections. He worked 6 days a week. He took part in some activities associated with the plumbers' union, went to sports events with some acquaintances, and for many years went to a gym. "I kept busy so I wouldn't feel so lonely." It appeared that Mr. Holden's interpersonal difficulties were larger than a propensity to lose his temper. He said that he generally felt awkward with other people, didn't know how to start a conversation or keep it going, and assumed that others looked down on him. "As I said at the beginning, I think it would be helpful to focus on how to better connect with others during our weekly meetings. With Charlie's move you feel like you have no one now. Let's put our heads together to think of ways in which you can make some acquaintances here at the nursing home." "Here? There are only old people here! What do I have in common with them?" "Well, would it hurt to try to find out?" Mr. Holden reluctantly agreed. On leaving the nursing home, the unit nurse took the therapist aside and said, "What have you been doing with Holden? He was actually less ornery this week!"

Session 8. The therapist was late to the session because of delay with another nursing home resident whom she was seeing. Mr. Holden stared at the therapist angrily. "Where have you been?" The therapist explained the reason for her delay. "I can see you're very annoyed," said the therapist. Mr.

Holden said he became convinced that the therapist was not coming that day and probably forgot about the appointment. Further discussion of the issue revealed that Mr. Holden thought the therapist had become less interested in him as she began to know him better. "That's not the case at all. I apologize for being late and will make every effort to be on time. I understand that this is a sensitive issue for you and that lateness contributed to difficulties with the aide." He said that as a child his father told him frequently that to be late was to show disrespect and when, as a child, he was late, his father sometimes beat him. The therapist encouraged him to speak more about his relationship with his father and he further revealed the details of a long history of ongoing physical abuse. The therapist empathized with the terrible difficulties he had to contend with as a child and said that it made a lot of sense that he would be sensitive to the way people treated him. "Would you agree that there are a lot of reasons that someone might be late that might not have anything to do with you?" He agreed and said that difficulties with people had been a problem for him throughout his adult life.

Session 9. The therapist conducted the HRSD, on which he had a score of 11. The therapist had intended to conduct the scale at Week 8 but waited because of the issue that arose over her lateness in visiting Mr. Holden. The therapist pointed out that his depressive symptoms were lower and that the nursing staff reported he seemed to have more energy and was gaining weight. He noted that the aide had been late twice in the past week but "I held my tongue" because another aide let him know that she would be late. He expressed appreciation for the therapist's visits and remarked, "I wish I would have met someone like you when I was younger." He said he had been thinking a lot about the therapist and asked if she were married. The therapist said that Mr. Holden appeared to be having some strong feelings about her. He acknowledged this and reiterated how lonely he was. "I appreciate that you have positive feelings for me. That's understandable given how lonely you've been. I think I can best be of help by working with you to make some connections with other people here in the nursing home." He said he understood but that "you can't take away the feelings that I have about you." Together they reviewed his relationships with nursing home residents and staff. He said that his roommate was "out of it" and he couldn't make a conversation with him. He avoided unit activities because he didn't like to spend time with "old people." The therapist encouraged him to spend some time with other residents in the TV room. He reluctantly agreed but said that other residents mainly wanted to watch soap operas. They discussed ways in which he might negotiate a change in the television channel in a manner that wouldn't offend other residents. They role-played a conversation with other residents. He said he would give it a try in the next week.

Session 10. Mr. Holden appeared somewhat brighter on the visit. He reported that he had gone to the TV room and, growing tired of the programming, asked, "Anybody here like sports?" Another resident responded, "I do!

There's a game on now." They successfully negotiated a channel change and during the course of the game he and the other resident, Allen, exchanged a few words about their common love of sports. "He wasn't a half bad guy." He and Allen acknowledged each other in the hallways several times and Allen told Mr. Holden that if they worked together as a "team" they could watch more sports. He said he learned that Allen was part of the card group on the unit. "So, might you think about joining?" asked the therapist. He said that he would think about it. Somewhat sheepishly he admitted that he had changed his colostomy bag once during the week when the aide was very late. She appeared upset about this but he said he contained his anger toward her. "We haven't discussed this before, Mr. Holden, but what has it been like for you to have the colostomy?" Mr. Holden seemed to wince at the question. He said that several years ago he had experienced months of rectal bleeding but had ignored it. Finally he went to the doctor and learned that he had advanced colon cancer. He admitted that he considered suicide when told that he would need to live with a colostomy and found the experience of the bag humiliating and embarrassing. "Who would want to know someone with a colostomy bag?" Mr. Holden said that the bag made him even more reluctant to engage with others in the nursing home and assumed that other residents were aware of it. "How would they know?" asked the therapist. He assumed that nursing staff told residents about the medical problems of fellow residents. "Has a staff person ever told you about other residents' medical problems?" He said no but argued that the nursing home was a small place and that word got around. The therapist conceded the possibility but said that, as a matter of policy, nursing staff were not to share medical information with other residents.

Session 11. Mr. Holden appeared somewhat more depressed. At first he said that there was no reason he should feel more depressed but later said that Allen had been taken to the hospital for medical problems. Nonetheless, he continued to go to the TV room and on several occasions was able to watch sports on television. "Do you know if Allen will be returning to the nursing home?" He said that he didn't know. "They don't tell you anything around here." The therapist gently remarked, "So the staff *doesn't* share medical information with residents!" He smiled and said, "You got me there." They laughed. "You have such a pretty smile," commented Mr. Holden. The therapist congratulated Mr. Holden for his efforts in going to the TV room and said that despite Allen's absence he appeared to be feeling less depressed. The therapist noted that with a decrease in his depressive symptoms it was likely easier for him to engage with people. She also congratulated him on his efforts to work better with the nursing aide. "She's not as bad as I thought." They continued discussion of past relationships and he expressed regrets that he had not made more efforts to connect with people. At the end of the session, Mr. Holden noted that he had recently seen his medical doctor and agreed to take antidepressant medication. "I think that was a good choice on your part. The medication should help you to feel even better."

Session 12. Mr. Holden was smiling when the therapist arrived. Allen had returned to the nursing home and, just prior to the therapist's arrival, the two men had a lively discussion about a recent baseball game. He expressed relief that Allen had returned to the home. Allen had invited him to join the floor card game. Mr. Holden said that at first he declined but later said that he would think about it. He expressed apprehension about entering the card group. Allen had said that the group played various card games, some of which Mr. Holden didn't know. He didn't like some of the other residents yet admitted he didn't really know them. Further, he was anxious about the fact that conversation did not come easily to him, especially with "strangers." Therapist and client discussed each of these concerns and explored options to deal with them. Perhaps Allen could teach Mr. Holden card games he didn't know prior to the card group meeting. One way to find out if he really liked the residents was to give the card group a try and make his decision afterward. Did the card group really require so much conversation? If he didn't say much at the beginning, perhaps others might take him to be a serious card player rather than as someone with little to say. "Why don't you go to the card game, see how things go, and then we can put our heads together next week if there are any problems." Mr. Holden agreed.

Session 13. Mr. Holden had attended the card group in the previous week. He said he felt awkward and had said little during the game, but was heartened at the end of the game when one of the members of the group said, "You're a pretty good card player." "It beats sitting in my room all day." The nursing aide who changed his colostomy bag told him that she would be leaving to take a job at a new nursing home. "Just when I was getting used to her," he said with some disappointment. Therapist and client discussed ways in which he could work with the new aide. "I guess I should tell her that I want to have my bag changed on time." They role-played an initial conversation with the aide. At first there was an angry, demanding tone to his communication, which the therapist pointed out. "I suspect that part of your anger has to do with the fact that you have a colostomy bag," noted the therapist. Mr. Holden said that he felt embarrassed and uncomfortable about having someone see his stoma. He said he would try his best to be "a gentleman."

Termination

Session 14. At the beginning of the session the therapist reminded Mr. Holden that two sessions remained. He was surprised and disappointed. He said that he did not recall that the therapy had been for 16 sessions. The therapist said that this had been discussed when they first met. He said he didn't remember this. The therapist realized that she had failed to periodically mention this to Mr. Holden as she typically did when conducting IPT. She apologized for failing to do this and wondered to herself whether she had not done this because of her own reluctance to end therapy with Mr. Holden. "I don't know what I'll do without you," he remarked. The therapist said that Mr. Holden was doing much better and that he appeared to be doing things pretty well by himself now. He said that he felt angry at the therapist. "Everyone leaves here. People die. Staff change. And now you're going." The therapist empathized with how hard it was to see so many people come and go. He worried that he would become depressed again. The therapist said that as therapy was ending, people often felt sad but this did not mean they were getting depressed. Mr. Holden said he wasn't convinced. The session ended somewhat awkwardly for both therapist and client.

Session 15. The therapist began the session by asking Mr. Holden whether he had further thoughts about ending therapy. He said that he continued to be disappointed about the end of therapy. He asked why therapy was only 16 sessions. The therapist said that this length of treatment generally was found to be helpful in reducing depression and helping people to better come to terms with the interpersonal problem that they were experiencing. He acknowledged that he was feeling better and that he was better connected to people in the nursing home. He asked if there might be a way for him to continue to see the therapist. The therapist said that she would think about this and that in the last session they would discuss it further. The session ended with a review of Mr. Holden's activities in the past week. He continued to spend time in the TV room and take part in the card group as well as visit with Allen.

Session 16. "Mr. Holden, I've got an idea. I run a group for residents of the nursing home on another floor. Although the group is only for residents of that floor I've checked with the nursing staff and they said that if you wanted to, you could join the group." Mr. Holden brightened. He expressed apprehension about meeting a new group of people but said that he would go. The therapist conducted the HRSD on which he had a score of 6, which is in the nondepressed range. "You've shown considerable improvement in your depression. At the beginning of therapy you had a score of 17 and now you have a score of 6. Furthermore, you are no longer in a major depression. As you recall, your depression was tied to the end of Charlie's visits. As you became more depressed you were more irritable, which made it even more difficult for you to deal with people, including the staff. During the time that we've worked together you patched things up with the aide, spent time in the TV room, met Allen, and took part in the card game. You've been brave in taking the risk to do these things. And now you're out of your depression." "Brave? Nobody ever said I was brave. My father said I was a coward." "Your father was wrong." The session ended with a discussion of the details of the group that Mr. Holden would be attending. "You're the best, doc."

Case Commentary

A review of past significant relationships with Mr. Holden was important as it revealed a troubled history of childhood abuse and poor interpersonal functioning in adult life. He was especially sensitive to rejection and the perception of disrespect from others and reacted with anger and withdrawal. The conflict that he initially had with the nursing aide who changed his colostomy bag likely reflected feelings of embarrassment and humiliation, negative racial attitudes, and inability to successfully negotiate differences. The end of his friend Charlie's visits increased feelings of isolation with subsequent depression. Interpersonal deficits were evident in his interactions with the therapist. Consistent with IPT strategies in the treatment of interpersonal deficits, differences with the therapist were discussed and negotiated in a way that helped him to build better social skills that he could use with other residents and staff. Repetitive problems in relationships were also reviewed with Mr. Holden. Communication analysis and role play further helped him to more productively engage with others. It was evident that Mr. Holden developed a strong attachment to the therapist—in psychodynamic parlance, a romantic transference. The expression of these feelings had to be diplomatically yet clearly addressed by the therapist so that she made clear that their relationship was a professional one and not a friendship. The therapist had not communicated to Mr. Holden the time-limited nature of the therapy during the course of treatment, perhaps because of her reluctance to end treatment with him. However, the therapist successfully transitioned Mr. Holden into a group where he could maintain a connection with the therapist in a context—group therapy—where he could further decrease social isolation and build social skills.

CONCLUDING COMMENTARY

The developmental transitions and challenges of later life may be especially disruptive for persons with limited interpersonal skills. These individuals may be very dependent on only one person, and that person's departure from their lives becomes a crisis. In light of the increasing dependence of older people on others for health-related problems, the absence of what Robert Weiss (1974) calls a *reliable alliance* can result in serious practical and emotional problems. For individuals with interpersonal deficits, nursing homes can be interpersonally demanding environments. Even for persons with a solid history of social relationships, life in a nursing home requires a new set of social skills that enable one to contend with dependence on staff and interactions with other residents, many of whom are experiencing physical or cognitive infirmities (Molinari, 2000). For those older persons with interpersonal deficits, nursing home life may feel overwhelming. Social withdrawal may be one means of handling these demands but it also increases feelings of loneliness and isolation and increases the risk for depression. For therapists working with frail residents of a nursing home—residents who see so many people come and go—feelings of protectiveness toward the client by the therapist are often elicited. As noted earlier, persons with interpersonal deficit typically require ongoing psychotherapeutic assistance beyond 16 weeks of IPT. Yet, within those 16 weeks, most clients demonstrate reduction of depressive symptoms and movement in the direction of the formation of new relationships. The therapist must be mindful of repetitive patterns that are reenacted within the therapeutic relationship as well as emotional attachments that may develop toward the therapist. Evidence of repetitive and attachment behaviors can be used by the therapist to help the client to better understand and change interpersonal behavior with others.

10

TERMINATION

In IPT, ending treatment is discussed from the beginning. As noted in chapter 5 (this volume), in the initial sessions, the therapist informs the client about the structure, frequency, and duration of therapy. The therapist provides a rationale for the length of treatment, explaining that 16 weeks of interpersonal psychotherapy (IPT) has been found to be effective in significantly reducing depressive symptoms for most individuals. Throughout IPT it is useful to intermittently remind the client of the number of remaining sessions. The eighth session, which is when we recommend administering a midtreatment depression inventory, is a particularly good time to note remaining sessions. Even when regular reminders are made of remaining sessions, some clients express some surprise when treatment comes to a close. The end of therapy is sometimes met with sadness. Nonetheless, most older adults we have treated with IPT have little difficulty ending psychotherapy. One of our IPT students suggested that the relative ease of older adults in ending IPT resulted from a lifetime of experience with endings. We also believe that ending therapy is not a problem for many because most older clients we have treated with IPT show significant improvement in depressive symptoms and ability to handle the problems that brought them to therapy. The chief question the therapist must deal with is whether the client should continue therapy beyond 16 sessions. This issue has gained increasing importance for therapists treating older adults since the publication of findings from the University of Pittsburgh maintenance treatment studies. As discussed in chapter 4 (this volume), investigators found that maintenance IPT and medication significantly reduced the likelihood of recurrence of depression in older adults with recurrent major depression (Reynolds et al., 1999).

EXPLICIT DISCUSSION OF TERMINATION

As is evident from the IPT outline (see Exhibit 10.1) and the illustrative clinical cases, formal discussion of termination begins in the 14th session and continues in the remaining IPT sessions. Although the issue of termination is raised in the 14th session, we usually find that most of the discussion of termination occurs in the 15th and 16th sessions. When the therapist anticipates that termination is going to be more difficult for a given client, all three termination sessions should be sharply focused on this topic.

ACKNOWLEDGMENT THAT TERMINATION IS A TIME OF GRIEVING

For most of our older clients, *sadness* rather than *grief* perhaps best captures the feeling. A special bond typically develops between therapist and client as they candidly discuss and address problems. For some older adults, the therapeutic relationship may be the first in which they have been able to talk about life issues without social constraints or considerations. In a generation in which the ethos often was "keep family business within the family," psychotherapy offers a unique opportunity. Almost always clients have feelings about the therapist. Within many psychodynamic psychotherapies, these feelings are interpreted as transference and used therapeutically. As previously noted, this is not the case in IPT. However, during termination, feelings about and attitudes toward the therapist may emerge. Some comments we have heard include the following: "I wish I had a daughter like you." "It's hard to believe a young person could understand the problems of an old person like me." "If I were forty years younger, I'd ask you out on a date." "You're my friend." These expressions are acknowledged and then the therapist usually moves the discussion to how the client feels about ending. Some clients avow that they have no problem with ending therapy and deny any feelings of sadness. This may be the case but it is important for the therapist to pursue the discussion of termination. Some clients are surprised to find that they do indeed have feelings about ending. Psychoeducation about the end of treatment can be useful. "It is not uncommon that people ending therapy have some feelings of sadness about the end." "Some people

tervention, with subsequent improvement of sleep and mood. Another client refused antidepressant medication at the beginning of IPT but agreed to take it when her symptoms did not improve at the end of IPT. Her depressive symptoms improved following a course of antidepressant medication. Mental health care professionals need to acknowledge to themselves, however, that some clients do not respond or only partially respond to existing psychotherapeutic or pharmacological interventions for depression. Nonetheless, all available options should be explored for those who do not respond to standard treatments for depression.

CONTINUATION/MAINTENANCE

As noted in chapter 4 (this volume), results from the University of Pittsburgh study attest to the importance of continuation and maintenance treatments for older adults with recurrent major depression (Reynolds et al., 1999). Since publication of those findings we have been more likely to provide maintenance IPT to older adults who have successfully completed acute IPT.

As discussed above, for clients who have only partially responded to IPT, continuation of weekly therapy for a determined length of time may be useful to ascertain whether further treatment will bring the desired outcomes. For clients who have significantly improved, some might continue into maintenance IPT. However, acute IPT treatment should be clearly demarcated from maintenance treatment. Even if it appears quite clear to the therapist that IPT treatment should continue, the termination phase of IPT should be completed. One reason is that the therapist should not prejudge what the client wants. This runs counter to IPT's stance that the client needs to explore all options and choose for him- or herself the one that seems best. It can be disheartening for a client who intends to end IPT—as has been originally agreed—to be directly or indirectly told that therapy should continue. For those clients who enter maintenance IPT, the last phase of acute treatment effectively becomes termination of acute treatment. During this final phase of acute IPT there is an opportunity to take stock of things and determine where treatment will likely go in the future.

For whom is maintenance treatment indicated? Research indicates that older adults with recurrent major depression, especially those for whom the problem area is interpersonal dispute, should continue with monthly IPT (Miller, Frank, Cornes, Houck, & Reynolds, 2003; Reynolds et al., 1999). In our clinical practice today, most clients with recurrent major depression who have improved with acute treatment continue in monthly maintenance therapy for about 6 months, at which time a decision is made whether to continue individual IPT. Clients who continue to have notable residual symptoms or active interpersonally relevant difficulties at the end of acute IPT will be tapered to twice monthly IPT and, if things improve, monthly IPT. If there is sustained improvement, IPT will end. If during the course of monthly IPT acute problems develop, we increase the frequency of sessions. Some clients who have completed IPT have returned several years later for another course of treatment related to a new problem area or exacerbation of the problem area that originally brought them into treatment. We sometimes refer clients who have completed a course of maintenance IPT to group psychotherapy.

In a maintenance form of IPT, the fundamental principles that guided acute IPT are used. Issues and lessons learned from acute IPT need to be integrated into maintenance sessions. "Do you remember how you were successful in handling the dispute with your daughter? Might some of the things you tried with her work with your son?" Reiteration of IPT psychoeducational messages is important: Depression is an illness; depression impairs ability to function; depression is a treatable illness; and interpersonally relevant events affect mood.

It is important to note that results from other studies of the course and outcome of depression in younger and older adults are cautionary about vulnerability of people treated for an acute episode of depression to future episodes (Cole & Bellavance, 1997; Reynolds, Alexopoulos, Katz, & Lebowitz, 2001). After treatment of the acute episode, many continue to have depressive symptoms. Most individuals who have had one episode of major depression will have another. One of the reasons for less than optimal outcomes or recurrence is that many clients do not receive adequate doses of antidepressant medication (Keller et al., 1982). We suspect that another reason is that they do not receive psychotherapy when needed or receive psychotherapeutic interventions that are not focused (Wei, Sambamoorthi, Olfson, Walkup, & Crystal, 2005). In clinical practice, practitioners know that the situation is even more complicated. Clinical studies often have clients who are not representative of clients in community practice. Community-treated older adults are more likely to have less clean, more complicated cases in which there are more medical and psychiatric comorbidities (notably personality disorders) than those in research studies, including IPT studies. Those who provide psychological services to older adults in nursing homes often confront some of the most complex cases, such as medically frail, cognitively impaired, older people with depression (Molinari, 2000). Clinicians are quick to point out these cases when we conduct IPT workshops. Our profession is challenged to further develop or refine existing treatments that take account of these issues. That being said, all mental health care professionals should strive to offer in an age-sensitive manner psychotherapeutic and pharmacological treatments that have evidence for their efficacy. We believe that, on the basis of our clinical experience, use of IPT with many older adults with depression maximizes therapeutic outcomes.

FURTHER COMMENTARY ON TERMINATION ISSUES
IN CLINICAL CASES

As the clinical cases discussed in chapters 5 through 9 illustrate, most older clients do not have significant problems ending IPT. Most felt some sadness about the anticipated end of treatment. Some clients experienced apprehension about the end of therapy that they misinterpreted as a return of depressive symptoms. The termination phase of IPT was most challenging for those with interpersonal deficits. Given these individuals' paucity of relationships, the therapist can become a central figure in their lives even during a brief treatment. Strong feelings of attachment can develop toward the therapist. In light of the propensity of persons with interpersonal deficits to misinterpret relationship issues, feelings and thoughts related to the planned ending need to be carefully addressed as the acute phase of IPT comes to an end. Rachel Greenberg, the woman with scoliosis and whose mother died, wondered whether the end of therapy was a way to get rid of her as a patient. Bob Holden, the man in the nursing home, saw the planned end of therapy as a rejection of him—a perception aided by the therapist's own reluctance to remind Mr. Holden during the middle sessions that the therapy would end.

Therapy did not continue beyond 16 weeks for the two clients for whom grief was the problem focus, Mrs. Johnson and Mr. O'Brien. Both had successfully dealt with the grief and associated interpersonal disputes with a concurrent reduction in depressive symptoms. Neither expressed a strong interest in continuing therapy. If there had been residual problems, the therapist would likely have seen these patients in maintenance treatment until problems and symptoms further improved. Mrs. Ryan and Mrs. Hernandez were the interpersonal role dispute clients. Treatment did not continue for Mrs. Ryan. However, in view of research findings on the usefulness of maintenance IPT, particularly for those recurrently older adults with depression (Reynolds et al., 1999), today we probably would have continued her in monthly IPT for a few months. Monthly sessions could have been used to monitor the status of the dispute with Mrs. Ryan's sister and, if difficulties arose, support her use of productive communication and problem-solving skills. In light of her long history of domestic abuse, it seemed prudent for Mrs. Hernandez to receive ongoing mental health care. At the end of acute treatment, she was seen in twice then once monthly IPT until she moved to Puerto Rico. If she had not moved, we would likely have continued her in monthly IPT for an indefinite period.

The two role-transition clients, May Barton and Cal Lewis, received additional services following the end of acute IPT. Mrs. Barton went to a support group for caregivers of relatives of dementia. It is worth noting that several years later Mrs. Barton contacted the therapist when her husband moved into a nursing home—another caregiving-related transition that was associated with depressive and anxiety symptoms for her. Another course of IPT was conducted with her around this new transition. Mr. Lewis was seen in maintenance IPT twice a month for 2 months and then monthly for another 6 months at which time treatment ended. Psychotherapeutic treatment continued for Rachel Greenberg and Bob Holden, the two clients with interpersonal deficits. Continued treatment is generally recommended for such clients (Weissman, Markowitz, & Klerman, 2000). Even though depressive symptoms decreased and these clients expanded their social worlds, both needed ongoing support. Ms. Greenberg had another 16-week course of IPT, which was reduced to monthly IPT. Eventually she transitioned into group psychotherapy. Mr. Holden completed individual IPT and then entered a group run by the therapist.

In sum, the advantage of time-limited therapy is that it can sharply focus psychotherapeutic resources on a life problem with clearly delineated goals within a specific time frame. Brevity of treatment makes each session important and makes both therapist and client think about how to best use therapeutic time. An end to treatment is an opportunity to take stock of therapeutic progress (or the lack thereof) and feelings about ending. Time-limited therapy has not been without its critics who, among a variety of concerns, complain that time limits are artificially imposed and reflect the constraints of research studies rather than realities of actual clinical practice (Levant, 2004). Solid evidence of high rates of recurrence in depression has challenged researchers to find way to reduce recurrence. One approach to reduce recurrence is to make sure that persons with depression are on adequate doses of antidepressant medication. Another approach for those with recurrent depression has been maintenance psychotherapies for depression. IPT was originally developed as a psychotherapy that would end for all who took part in it. IPT in the treatment of acute depression now has a companion treatment—maintenance IPT. For those who continue into maintenance IPT, the termination phase is focused less on feelings of loss of the therapist (who will likely remain as the maintenance IPT therapist) than on a review of treatment progress and plans for future treatment. Future research will determine the optimal duration of maintenance IPT. As always, practicing clinicians will need to use their best judgment about duration of therapy for individual clients.

11

ISSUES IN IMPLEMENTATION OF INTERPERSONAL PSYCHOTHERAPY WITH OLDER ADULTS

Over the years, we have supervised psychiatrists, psychologists, social workers, paraprofessionals, and graduate students conducting interpersonal psychotherapy (IPT) with varied age groups including older adults. Most supervisees develop a fairly good grasp of IPT after completion of one supervised case. All of them benefit from supervision of one or two additional cases to solidify IPT skills. Although formal standards for training individuals in IPT are only now being codified, most research studies have required that an individual complete an introductory course, conduct three audio- or videotaped IPT cases, and receive weekly supervision for each case. As discussed in chapter 3 (this volume), rating scales for IPT treatment fidelity have been used in studies; and therapists who faithfully conduct IPT generally have better therapeutic outcomes than do those with less fidelity (see Frank & Spanier, 1995, for review). There are ongoing discussions within the International Society of Interpersonal Psychotherapy about what best constitutes substantive training in IPT and whether it makes sense to develop a formal mechanism for accreditation. Among psychology externs, interns, and postdoctoral fellows supervised for IPT with older adults conducted by Hinrichsen, clinical outcomes for their cases were comparable to those of trained staff (Hinrichsen, 2004). In this chapter we discuss some common problems that supervisees have in implementing IPT. We also discuss some problematic clinical situations with older clients and offer suggestions for handling them.

GENERAL ISSUES

The therapist does not believe that substantive therapeutic work can be achieved in 16 sessions. Some novice IPT therapists have doubts about what can be achieved in this or other brief therapies.

Various problems and their associated clinical goals require different kinds of treatment. The primary goals of IPT are significant reduction in depressive symptoms and improvement in the designated interpersonal problem area(s). These are important yet circumscribed goals. IPT does not target fundamental characterological change. IPT practitioners assume (with some research evidence to support the assumption) that success in dealing with current life problems may help the client contend with future interpersonally relevant difficulties. Knowledge of research-verified success of IPT along with positive outcomes in actual clinical practice builds the therapist's conviction that IPT is an adaptable and useful treatment. (See chaps. 3 and 4, this volume, for a brief review of relevant research outcomes and also Weissman, Markowitz, & Klerman, 2000, for more detailed reviews of studies.) This conviction will be communicated directly and indirectly to IPT clients, helping to counteract feelings of hopelessness evident in individuals with depression.

The therapist believes that IPT's illness conceptualization of depression is not a useful one. Some nonphysician mental health care therapists have difficulty accepting an illness model of major depression. Some feel that mental health has generally been medicalized in a way that does injustice to the complexity of life problems. The *DSM–IV* psychiatric nosology is a simplistic way of characterizing human problems. Depression is less a psychiatric illness than a response to life problems.

Hinrichsen, a psychologist, and Clougherty, a psychiatric social worker, find the illness model of major depression a compelling one. The functional impairment caused by major depression is as or more severe than that caused by many major medical illnesses (Wells et al., 1989). Major depression is associated with physiological, cognitive, and affective symptoms and increases risk for mortality. Brain scans now document unique changes associated with major depression in select areas of the brain and that treatment with antidepressant medication or psychotherapy appears to normalize these changes (A. L. Brody et al., 2001). The condition is recurrent. Major depression damages social relationships (Joiner, 2000). Major depression is certainly a unique illness that attests to the complex interplay between the brain and environment. IPT strategically uses the notion of depression as illness in treatment as a rationale for temporary reduction of role responsibilities and self-blame for depression-related disability.

The therapist wonders how much change is possible for older adults. Some therapists feel that because older people have well-established patterns of living or long-term problems, they are unlikely to be responsive to psychotherapy. Some older adults seem to have so many problems—physical, social, psychiatric—that a short-term treatment is seen as too little, too late.

As discussed in chapter 2 (this volume), a solid body of research shows that older adults with depression benefit from psychotherapy and medication in a way that is not markedly different from how adults benefit. Therapeutic pessimism about older people usually reflects a lack of information, lack of experience with older people and those with health problems, and personal unease with aging.

The therapist is pessimistic about prospects for change in a person with severe or recurrent depression. Some clients have long histories of depression or are in a current episode of protracted, severe depression. These facts make the therapist wary about prospects for change.

Research studies demonstrate that depression is contagious—that is, those living with a person with depression are more likely to subsequently experience depressive symptoms than those who do not live with a person with depression. Powerful interpersonal forces are at work that can create therapeutic pessimism even among experienced clinicians. We are reminded of a middle-aged former IPT client with severe depression who had at least 10 episodes of major depression, 3 marriages, 15 jobs, and a history of alcoholism. His initial presentation made us wonder how much improvement he could achieve in a brief therapy. The therapist worked closely with a highly skilled psychopharmacologist and the client had an excellent clinical outcome. No doubt this man would require ongoing mental health care throughout his life. Nonetheless, a course of acute IPT helped him deal with pressing interpersonal problems and depression. Clinical outcomes should not be prejudged even in very difficult cases.

The therapist does not maintain adherence to the IPT outline. Some therapists have problems keeping therapy within the goals of IPT. It is imperative that before beginning IPT with a first case, the therapist completely read the IPT manual (i.e., Weissman et al., 2000) and books and articles relevant to the use of IPT with a particular problem or population. It is useful to reread sections of the book(s) as therapy progresses into different phases (e.g., reread the termination session section prior to commencing therapy). Just prior to beginning a session, it is helpful to quickly review the IPT outline that pertains to the phase of therapy that is being conducted and the established problem area(s). For example, if the focus of IPT is interpersonal disputes, the goals and strategies for that problem area should be reviewed. During the course of each session, the therapist can mentally relate the topic being dis-cussed to a goal, strategy, or technique. In addition to keeping therapy on track, this mental effort helps novice therapists to consolidate their under-standing of the elements of IPT. If, in the course of therapy, it is not clear to the therapist how a particular topic is relevant to IPT, the therapy is likely off track. One rule of thumb is that the therapist ought to be able to link in his or her mind the reasons for any discussion occurring during a session to the problem area. At the end of the full, 16-week acute treatment of the first IPT client, it may be helpful to reread treatment manuals.

The therapist is uncomfortable taking a directive role. Therapists are some-times reluctant to redirect clients. They may feel that interrupting the flow of the client's verbalizations may harm the therapeutic alliance relationship. It feels disrespectful to interrupt or redirect an older person.

Although there is considerable latitude for the client to discuss a vari-ety of issues, IPT does operate with identified goals tied to specific problems. Sometimes clients stray from that framework. Most older adults expect the therapist to take the lead in therapeutic sessions. We also find that keeping things on track from the beginning sends a clear message to the client about what topics are relevant to the treatment (in other words, they begin to be socialized into IPT therapy). Therapists trained in psychodynamic psycho-therapies are most likely to feel discomfort in taking the therapeutic lead. One supervisee with a very strong psychodynamic background told the su-pervisor, "I was trained to be very careful about pushing my own agenda with the client." "You're not pushing your agenda," replied the supervisor. "You're implementing a treatment plan supported by research and agreed upon by the client."

The therapist is not sure whether a potential client is a good candidate for IPT. Research studies attests to the versatility of IPT. The ideal training case is an older adult diagnosed with a fairly recent onset of major depression with a clearly identified interpersonal problem area. In clinical practice with older adults, we use IPT for older adults with major depression (single or recurrent episode) and adjustment disorder (with depressive symptoms or mixed anxi-ety and depression). We have also treated a small number of older adults with dysthymia or a major depression and dysthymia (i.e., double depres-sion). Clients with dysthymia almost always require more than 16 weeks of IPT (Markowitz, 1998). Some of our clients have partially remitted major depression and are referred from an inpatient service or partial psychiatric hospital program. If a client has evidence of cognitive impairment, we want to make sure that the client will likely be able to recall the general purpose of therapy and be able to make efforts independently between sessions to ad-dress interpersonal issues. We believe that individuals with marked charac-ter pathology (most notably, borderline personality disorder) are best treated with other modalities (e.g., dialectical behavior therapy) although at the time of this writing a pilot research study is examining the usefulness of a modified form of IPT for persons with borderline personality disorder. When the most prominent symptom is anxiety, we often find that cognitive–behavioral therapy is the treatment of choice. The bottom line is that IPT seems most appropriate for a generally cognitive intact individual who is depressed and who has an interpersonal issue relevant to one of the four IPT problem areas.

The client has problems focusing on the relevant problem area(s). Some older clients have difficulty focusing on relevant therapeutic issues. They discuss issues other than those IPT issues that were agreed upon in the initial sessions. They may be tangential and circumstantial. For example, a discussion of a current problem with a spouse may quickly transition into a detailed account of early courtship and what it was like living during World War II.

Maintaining therapeutic focus is not an issue unique to older adults or to IPT. Lack of focus, however, becomes particularly problematic when the number of sessions is set in advance and the therapist (and also the client) may have a feeling that precious time is being wasted. It is important to raise this issue as soon as it develops. At first this can be done gently. "I'd like to return to discussion of the problem with your husband. Given our limited time, I think it is most useful to focus on this." For clients who continue to have difficulties focusing, it is useful to directly address the problem. If, in the course of a session, the client becomes tangential, the therapist might say, "I'd like to stop you now to talk about something that I think is important. As we've discussed, it seems like you have problems staying on one topic. Did you notice that this just happened again?" If problems persist, further discussion is warranted. The therapist and client might negotiate how the therapist can respectively yet firmly alert the client to the need for topic redirection. One client asked the therapist to raise her hand when she strayed from the topic. Often this hand signal provoked laughter for both and then redirection. Most clients are aware of their tendency to stray ("Oh yes, my husband says that I do that") and are willing to work collaboratively with the therapist.

There are varied reasons why some older clients have problems maintaining focus. Cognitive researchers have noted the phenomenon of off-target verbosity in older adults and suggest that changes in the aging brain make it more difficult for some older adults to remain on track verbally (Arbuckle, Nohara-LeClair, & Pushkar, 2000). Some older adults have a history of difficulty focusing on life problems. Movement away from a problem may be an unconscious psychological strategy to avoid an issue that raises anxiety. The therapist's effort to focus the client may help the client to gain clarity about the issue of concern as well as possible options. We occasionally have clients who have problems maintaining therapeutic focus because they have early symptoms of dementia. Although cognitive impairment is not necessarily a bar to psychotherapy with older adults, therapeutic memory aids such as written summaries of sessions, regular restatements of central therapeutic issues, and use of family members are often helpful therapeutic adjuncts. Only recently have researchers turned their attention to understanding how to successfully adapt psychotherapies for older adults with cognitive problems. In rare cases, it may be necessary to discontinue IPT and use a less focused, more supportive approach.

The client is late or misses appointments. Attendance problems are not specific to IPT. However, the issue may be more problematic than it is in long-term treatments because absences reduce the total amount of time in IPT. Attendance problems need to be directly addressed from the beginning. If problems are not addressed, the client may assume that it is acceptable to be late or cancel appointments. When visiting medical care providers, some older adults routinely wait a half hour or more beyond their appointment time before they are seen. Those unfamiliar with psychotherapy may assume that the therapist will also be late in starting appointments. It is useful to understand why the client is having attendance problems and use these difficulties as an opportunity to generate options and possible solutions to the problem. Sometimes attendance problems develop because the client is ambivalent about continuing treatment. This possibility may need to be raised and addressed, and a decision made by the client about continuing treatment.

The client feels hopeless that things can change. Feelings of hopelessness are common in depression. In the initial sessions, the therapist educates the client about this fact along with the fact that feelings of hopelessness will decrease as the client improves. "It is difficult to see that things will get better when you are in the midst of a major depression. The facts are on our side—that is, the majority of people with depression will improve from treatment." During the course of treatment the client may express disappointment that depression is not improving or that adequate progress is not being made in the problem area. If the therapist believes that progress indeed is being made, he or she will tell this to the client. For other clients, the therapist concurs with the client's assessment that there is little change in symptoms or the identified problem. In either case, the therapist underscores that hopelessness is a key symptom of depressive illness and that it is understandable that the client would be prone to view things negatively and hopelessly. As previously noted, the therapist needs to be vigilant about adopting a similarly pessimistic view.

THE INITIAL SESSIONS

The therapist feels there is too much to cover in three sessions. Some mental health professionals use the early weeks or even months of therapy to get a detailed developmental history. A 3-week review of issues seems superficial to the therapist.

Concern about the length of the initial sessions often reflects larger concerns about how much can be accomplished in a time-limited treatment. A well-organized and goal-directed therapist can usually adequately cover the content of initial sessions. It is helpful to keep in mind that information gleaned in the initial sessions provides a broad overview of relevant diagnostic and interpersonal issues. In the middle sessions, much more time will be devoted to issues deemed important to treatment. Therapists sometimes veer off course in the initial sessions when they get sidetracked with issues that are not pertinent to IPT. Or, they devote too much time to an in-depth discussion of a relevant issue that should be explored in detail in the middle sessions.

The therapist finds it difficult to conduct the interpersonal inventory in one session. There may be times when an inexperienced IPT therapist may need more than one session to complete the interpersonal inventory. With practice most should be able to accomplish this task in one session.

It may be helpful to explain the framework for the interpersonal inventory to the patient. "During this session, we are going to discuss important relationships in your life. We will not go into depth about each of these relationships as I want to get a general sense of the important people in your life. Therefore, we will talk for no more than 5 or 10 minutes about each person." It is sometimes tempting to spend considerable time reviewing details of a relationship that will likely be the focus of treatment. However, there will be plenty of time to do that in the middle sessions. We tell IPT supervisees that we want to gain a broad view of interpersonal relationships to (a) see if there is an interpersonally relevant area that could be a focus of treatment but was not apparent from information the client initially provided, (b) get a sense of the general pattern of relationships with others, and (c) identify any past interpersonal issues that might be relevant to current problems. A particular challenge in conducting the interpersonal inventory with older adults is that they have lived many years. It is important to ascertain whether there are interpersonally relevant early-life issues. Examples of these include illness or death of parents, separation from parents, and early-life trauma. For those who are widowed, it is important to get a sense of the kind of relationship the client had with the deceased. We find that the questions listed in the IPT outline for the interpersonal inventory are useful ones and we encourage supervisees to use them.

The client has several relevant problems areas or multiple life problems and the therapist is not clear where to focus. Some clients have especially complicated lives and it may be hard for the therapist to decide what may be the most profitable area on which to focus.

It is helpful to discern which interpersonally relevant problem was most closely tied to the onset of depression. Also, which interpersonal problem is of most concern to the client? Because the therapy is brief, it is not possible to therapeutically address more than one or two major problem areas. If in doubt, the therapist should ask the client which problem(s) would be most helpful to focus on in therapy. During the middle sessions other life issues may arise but, on the whole, the therapist needs to maintain focus on the agreed upon problem area(s).

The therapist is unsure which of the four interpersonal problem areas best suits the client's problem. The therapist may wonder whether an older adult transitioning into the role of dementia caregiver might also warrant grief as a problem area.

We find that the IPT problems areas are defined broadly enough so that they encompass most interpersonally relevant issues that clients bring to therapy. For beginning therapists, however, the breadth of definition can create confusion about which problem area is most appropriate for a given client's issue. One confusion is that feelings of loss or mourning are part of interpersonal disputes and role transitions. Novice IPT therapists often wonder whether grief should be an additional area. We tell supervisees that a more careful reading of the manual indicates that the grief problem area is reserved for those with complicated bereavement. Supervisees may also wonder whether a client with grief may also warrant role transitions as a secondary area as the client will be making a transition to the role of widowed person. However, transitioning into a life without the deceased is an integral goal of grief and does not require another problem area. Sometimes supervisees ask whether persons with interpersonal disputes should have interpersonal deficits as a second problem area. Their rationale is that because the client is having problems negotiating a conflict he or she must have an interpersonal deficit. We emphasize that the problem area of interpersonal deficits is reserved for individuals with marked problems in forming or sustaining relationships. Part of the confusion is that the development of relevant interpersonal skills is a strategy in each of the four problem areas.

As noted in earlier chapters, we find that role transitions is a problem area where many late-life problems can be accommodated. Examples include transitioning into the caregiving role, the role of a person with health problems, a new residence or community, retirement, and parenting responsibilities.

A clear formulation and plan are not given to the client. The therapist may not pull together elements of the initial sessions into a clear statement of the problem and plan for treatment.

We find it especially important that a succinct problem statement be given to the client at the end of the third session. "Now I'd like to tell you what I think." With this statement, the therapist can pull together all the elements of the initial sessions in a clear way. "Now I'd like you to tell me what you think about what I've said." With this, the therapist asks whether he or she has correctly understood the client's concerns. "This is what I'm recommending for treatment." The therapist offers a plan. "Let me know if this makes sense to you." The therapist asks for client assent to proceed with a treatment plan. This problem and treatment formulation can be repeated in the middle sessions and also in the termination phase when progress in treatment is reviewed. Repetition is often very useful in psychotherapy.

The therapist forgets to adequately explain the treatment contract. Many beginning therapists forget to explain the duration of treatment, emphasize the importance of the client's attendance, or get the client's agreement about the focus of treatment in the initial sessions.

The therapist has a difficult time transitioning from the initial to the intermediate sessions. The tasks of the initial session are fairly well outlined. The goals and strategies of the middle sessions are more global and leave some therapists wondering how to proceed.

We believe one advantage of IPT is that unlike some psychotherapies, the specific content of each session is not outlined. The broad goals and strategies of IPT allow a great deal of therapeutic flexibility. For novice IPT therapists, that flexibility can be intimidating because they worry whether they are adhering to the treatment structure. As noted above, one of the best ways to remain treatment adherent is to review the IPT outline and continue to ask oneself, "How is this discussion relevant to the IPT goals and strategies for this problem area?"

THE INTERMEDIATE SESSIONS

The therapist drops discussion of depressive symptoms or depressive illness. Once there has been a discussion of depression in the initial sessions, some therapists rarely refer to it thereafter.

On a regular basis the therapist should inquire about the status of depressive symptoms. "How's the depression?" Although we recommend conducting a depression rating scale at the beginning, middle, and end of IPT, it can be done more often. This information helps to mark therapeutic progress and provides an opportunity to link interpersonally relevant events from the prior week to an increase or decrease in symptoms. It can be helpful to ask about only those depressive symptoms from a depression rating scale that the client reported in the prior week's session. When the client reports difficulties in functioning, the therapist can remind the client that depression is the likely reason. Repeating educational information about depression from the initial sessions can be helpful. Continued discussion of depression conveys to the client that the therapist understands the problem. "Depression is such a terrible illness because it makes it so hard to get through the day. But we're working together so that you will be out of this episode."

The therapist is too quick to provide advice to the client. Some clients have problems coming up with ideas and the therapist offers suggestions without first exploring options.

Giving suggestions to clients may be perfectly appropriate. When clients are stuck, however, it is useful to encourage them to try to identify options themselves. An idea that comes from the client builds the client's confidence that options can be self-generated. When a client does not feel that options can be generated, the therapist might ask: "What have you done in a situation like this before?" "What would other people have done?" "Have you had friends in a similar situation?" If the client continues to have difficulties in identifying options, ask the client to think about the issue in the coming week. If the client is still stuck, the therapist may offer ideas and ask what the client thinks about them.

For some clients with grief as the problem area, the therapist may be reluctant to focus sessions on the deceased because the topic seems too painful to the client. The therapist may be the only person with whom the client can discuss the loss. The therapist needs to sensitively, empathetically, and firmly encourage the client to discuss the loss. For reluctant clients, the therapist may comment, "I know you don't feel ready for this discussion now and we will put it aside for the rest of the session. However, we will need to get back to it in the next session."

For clients with interpersonal disputes, the therapist wonders whether it is appropriate to include the party to the dispute in sessions. The answer is a qualified yes. It can be very helpful to include the other person in one or two sessions. The therapist can get a much more tangible sense of how the client relates to the other party. Inclusion of the other party seems appropriate if the client is interested and the other party assents. Planning in advance for the joint meeting is recommended. A joint meeting might be a good place where the client can practice better communication skills. In the next session, following the joint meeting, it will be helpful to give the client feedback on how he or she interacted with the other party.

The therapist fails to remind the client of remaining sessions. It is only toward the end of therapy that the therapist indicates that treatment is coming to a close.

Every few sessions it is useful to note the session number. "This is our 10th session, with six remaining." Reminders to the client of remaining sessions can motivate some to make more active efforts to change the interpersonal issue of concern. For clients who are likely going to have problems ending acute IPT, regular reminders make this process easier.

TERMINATION

The therapist assumes psychotherapy will continue beyond 16 weeks. Often novice IPT therapists find it difficult to terminate therapy. Sometimes shortly after beginning the termination phase they will make off-hand remarks such as "We'll be ending IPT but I think we can probably continue" or "Although we're coming to the end of therapy, I suspect you'd like to continue."

Therapists with little experience in conducting time-limited psychotherapies often are uncomfortable with terminating therapy after 16 weeks. They subjectively feel they are abandoning the person. Termination may be especially difficult for some therapists working with older adults. Older adults frequently have a variety of ongoing late-life stressors—most notably, health concerns—that may or may not be related to depression. We remind our supervisees that a contract was made with the client at the beginning of treatment for 16 weeks of treatment. When indicated, this contract can be renegotiated but the therapist must not prejudge what the client wants. Directly or indirectly communicating that the client needs more treatment sends the message that he or she is not capable of handling life problems without psychotherapy. This message runs against the empowerment ethos of IPT. Research studies demonstrate, in fact, that offering more help to older adults than is wanted or needed can damage their self-esteem and sense of control (Newsom & Schulz, 1998). Some clients are disappointed and perplexed that the therapist assumes that they will continue psychotherapy beyond 16 weeks. They feel they have made progress ("Didn't the therapist say I was doing better?"), had expected to end treatment ("Wasn't I told this was 16 weeks?"), have other obligations ("Do you know how many doctor visits I have each week?"), and don't want to bear the expense of additional weekly psychotherapy sessions ("Do you know how much I put out each month for health care expenses?"). Some clients want to continue IPT even though they have done very well because they confuse sadness about ending with relapse of symptoms. When these termination issues are processed, most are comfortable with ending treatment. As discussed in chapter 10 (this volume), however, continuation of some form of treatment is indicated for some individuals—particularly those who have only partially responded to IPT, those with recurrent depression, or those with ongoing interpersonal disputes.

12

NEXT STEPS

A few years ago Hinrichsen called a beloved former psychotherapy supervisor who had retired and was living abroad. In the course of the conversation she asked, "Greg, how much psychotherapy do you do now?" He replied that psychotherapy with older adults was an important part of his professional work and that it was a source of personal and professional satisfaction. She commented, "I remember when you were a psychology intern. You were compassionate and well-intentioned but you needed a method. Did you find a method?" "Yes," he replied, "I found a method."

As noted in chapter 4 (this volume), in clinical work we have found that interpersonal psychotherapy (IPT) seems well-suited to the problems of older adults. IPT addresses interpersonal problems that commonly co-occur with depression, is well-received by most older adults, and appears to have good clinical outcomes with our older clients. As therapists, we think of IPT as less of a method than a conceptually coherent, empirically grounded, and flexibly applied set of goals, strategies, and techniques.

As noted earlier in this volume, when we conduct IPT workshops, seasoned professionals often tell us that they already use elements of IPT in their clinical work. Such comments are heartening to us because IPT is strongly informed by the clinical experience of Klerman and Weissman in the treatment of persons with depression. Other professionals sometimes ask how IPT is conceptually distinct from CBT and psychodynamic psychotherapy. We sometimes respond by citing Klerman, Weissman, Rounsaville, and Chevron's (1984) outline of differences between IPT and other psychotherapies. Or we review Weissman, Markowitz, and Klerman's (2000) summary of salient characteristics distinguishing IPT from other psychotherapies: time-limited, focused, primary discussion on current relationships, interpersonal, not focused on personality. Yet, IPT does share some similarities with psychodynamic psychotherapies (e.g., focus on underlying issues, repetitive patterns in relationships, selective attention to historical relationship) and cognitive–behavioral therapies (e.g., enlargement in scope of activities and involvements, change of expectations). The techniques used in IPT (e.g., exploration, clarification, encouragement of affect) are used in many other psychotherapies. Parochial battles among different schools of psychotherapy have softened in recent years as psychotherapy adherents honestly acknowledge the power of factors common among most psychotherapies to reduce psychiatric symptoms (Horvath, 1988). Also, there has been a move away from the one-size-fits-all approach taken by some therapeutic schools (i.e., my therapy can fix any problem) to an intellectual and research curiosity about which therapy works best for which problems.

Is a method really useful? We believe a conceptual frame benefits clinical work. After many years of providing psychotherapeutic services to older people, Hinrichsen found that IPT was a solid framework on which to hang many of the strategies and techniques he found that helped his older clients with depression. Clougherty similarly found that use of IPT strengthened the psychotherapeutic work she had been doing for many years. For both of us, IPT provided an overarching rationale for conceptualizing, prioritizing, and responding to the many issues that inevitably arise in conducting therapy. IPT was an avenue for meaningfully integrating a larger body of research on interpersonal issues and depression that is relevant to the therapeutic encounter. Clinical confidence was enhanced by the large body of research that supports the usefulness of IPT in the treatment of depression and other problems. What we like most about IPT is its central ethos of empowerment. "What are your options?" is the IPT mantra. That simple question conveys the conviction that there are always possible ways of responding to life's problems even when things look their darkest. Another comment we often make to patients is "That's your depression speaking." This response conveys an understanding that depression is a powerful illness that can negatively constrict thinking so much that the person with depression can hardly imagine a past or future time when life was or could be rewarding. The comment also conveys with it the message that most illnesses improve and we expect the client's depressive illness to improve too. Clougherty was privileged to take part in the first randomized, controlled clinical trial of psychotherapy in Uganda, the same IPT Uganda study cited in chapter 3 (this volume; Bolton et al., 2003). It was striking to her that a psychotherapy developed in America could be adapted to the culture of Uganda and applied with such great success. Of course, it is an empirical question whether other psychotherapies might have had similar success. Nonetheless, IPT's hopeful message was a helpful message in a non-Western culture.

That being said, much work remains. Though mental health professionals do a good job in the treatment of acute depression, many people have additional episodes of depression (Keller, Lavori, & Mueller, 1992; Reynolds et al., 2001). Practicing clinicians know this all too well and researchers have documented that reality. A minority of individuals do not or minimally respond to the treatment of acute depression. New antidepressant medications now exist. Though SSRIs have many fewer side effects than do the older generation of antidepressants (i.e., the tricyclic antidepressants), there is concern about weight gain and sexual dysfunction associated with SSRI use. Most primary care physicians neither adequately diagnose nor treat depression despite the fact that they prescribe the majority of psychotropic medications (Higgins, 1994). Treatments for late-life depression have improved in the past 20 years. Yet treatment of depression with antidepressants in older people is complicated by the much greater presence of health problems and associated use of medications for those medical problems than with younger persons (e.g., pharmacokinetics that differ between old and young, interactions among medications, greater sensitivity to side effects; Reynolds et al., 2001). Despite the demonstrated efficacy of psychotherapy, the mainstay in the treatment of depression in older adults as well as younger adults is medication. Antidepressant treatment of late-life depression without psychotherapy may be a reasonable course of action. Yet in light of strong research evidence that interpersonally relevant problems often precede depression and influence the course of depression in young and old, psychotherapy appears underused in older adults (Hinrichsen & Emery, 2005; Wei, Sambamoorthi, Olfson, Walkup, & Crystal, 2005). Despite the existence of cognitive impairment and dementia, particularly in the "oldest old" (i.e., persons 85 years and older), little research has examined the usefulness of psychotherapy for older adults with cognitive impairment. Psychologists who work in nursing homes report that psychotherapy is often useful even for older people with mild to moderate cognitive impairment (Molinari, 2000). Little empirical evidence exists to support or refute that observation. It is fortunate that several research studies of the usefulness of psychotherapy for older adults with cognitive impairment and depression are in development. Mark Miller (2004) at the University of Pittsburgh has adapted IPT for older adults with cognitive impairment and depression; Brian Carpenter and his colleagues at Washington University have developed an innovative psychotherapy for long-term care residents (Carpenter, Ruckdeschel, Ruckdeschel, & Van Haitsma, 2002); and Dimitris Kiosses at Weill Medical College of Cornell University is adapting problem-solving therapy for older people with cognitive deficits.

A definitive randomized clinical trial of IPT in the acute treatment of major depression in older adults remains to be conducted. The two studies that have been conducted in the treatment of acute depression in late life are basically pilot work (Rothblum, Sholomskas, Berry, & Prusoff, 1982; Sloane, Staples, & Schneider, 1985). The other relevant treatment study in medically ill older adults with depressive symptoms uses interpersonal counseling (IPC, the brief version of IPT; Mossey, Knott, Higgins, & Talerico, 1996). The irony is that acute treatment studies are much easier to conduct than are continuation/maintenance studies. Though data are limited for the usefulness of IPT in the acute treatment of depression, a rich set of findings is available from a large, well-designed study in the continuation/maintenance treatment of late-life depression. Among many findings, the continuation/maintenance study found that monthly sessions of IPT alone, medication alone, or the combination of IPT and medication reduced recurrence of major depression (Reynolds et al., 1999). The reader is invited to conduct the definitive IPT acute treatment study with older adults!

So, after reading this book, what do you do if you want to conduct IPT with older adults? As noted several times, read *Comprehensive Guide to Interpersonal Psychotherapy* (Weissman et al., 2000). *Comprehensive Guide* includes the original treatment manual and contains excellent summaries of research and applications of IPT to varied populations and problems. It is a clinically friendly book filled with very helpful case material. We encourage students we supervise in IPT to read the book in advance of their yearlong training and again at the end of the training. The reader of *Interpersonal Psychotherapy for Depressed Older Adults* will find that *Comprehensive Guide* consolidates what has been learned in reading this book.

For those who have little or no clinical experience with older adults, it is important that they become familiarized with geropsychology. The American Psychological Association's (APA's) "Guidelines for Psychological Practice With Older Adults" (APA, 2004) is a good starting place. Bob Knight's *Psychotherapy With Older Adults* (Knight, 2004) is highly recommended. Other bibliographic recommendations can be found in this book's Resources section. There are a variety of training workshops in geropsychology, some of which are listed on APA's Division 12, Section II (clinical geropsychology) Web site, http://www.geropsych.org. APA's Office on Aging also has a Web site (http://www.apa.org/pi/aging) with useful resources including those related to psychotherapy with older adults and practical suggestions related to billing Medicare.

Is formal supervision required to become proficient in IPT? We believe it is. This question and the answer raise a host of issues. For example, how do health professionals acquire new skills? Most states require ongoing continuing education activities as a condition of licensure and they are dutifully attended. No doubt many of these are excellent but, in our view, are more often updates on one or more dimension of clinical practice than opportunities to substantively acquire new skills. Both of the authors conduct full-day training workshops on IPT but do not believe that at the end of the workshop participants are proficient in IPT. Among geropsychologists who provide continuing education, there is ongoing discussion about how we can provide a meaningful set of continuing education activities related to geropsychology that incrementally build skills (Qualls, Segal, Norman, Niederehe, & Gallagher-Thompson, 2002). The issue of professional continuing education is especially relevant for practicing psychologists with no or limited experience in providing services to older adults who want to acquire geropsychology-related knowledge and skills. One admirable effort in this regard has been made by geropsychologist Sara Qualls, who began a yearly geropsychology training conference at the University of Colorado–Colorado Springs in 2005. Each year the conference addresses different topics that, in the aggregate, cover critical issues in the provision of clinical services to older people.

In some areas of the country, professional institutes provide ongoing, supervised training in mental health. Some institutes with which we are familiar specialize in psychoanalysis, family therapy, marital therapy, and cognitive–behavioral therapy. Participants take part in course work, receive clinical supervision of their work with clients, and are issued certificates at the end of program completion. Hinrichsen's home institution recently established the Committee for Empirically Supported Psychological Practices. The chief mission of the committee is the dissemination of empirically supported practices to fellow psychologists for use with clients across the age span through training workshops, individual supervision, and group supervision.

So where can training and supervision in IPT be obtained? IPT training workshops are offered by various individuals and institutions throughout the year. Workshops are sometimes advertised in professional publications. A good place to look is the Web site of the International Society for Interpersonal Psychotherapy (http://www.interpersonalpsychotherapy.org). These workshops will provide a good overview of IPT or the use of IPT with specific populations or problems. Finding an IPT supervisor may be more challenging. Despite the large number of studies that have demonstrated the efficacy of IPT, the treatment is not widely disseminated. Therefore, it will likely be more difficult to locate a geographically proximate supervisor than it would be for other modalities (e.g., cognitive–behavioral therapy). Nonetheless, if a prospective IPT supervisor is not within driving distance, supervision may be conducted by telephone. Usually the supervisee audio- or videotapes sessions and sends them to the supervisor for comment. (With the advent of digital tape recorders, sessions can now be e-mailed.)

How much supervision is required to obtain proficiency in IPT? The current IPT supervision paradigm comes from research studies that have required three supervised cases. Some have questioned whether three cases are necessary to obtain proficiency in IPT. Debate also exists about the wisdom of establishing a formal certification in IPT: Will certification ensure high-quality IPT or discourage professionals from using the therapy? We are mindful that obtaining formal supervision in IPT can be an expensive proposition. Supervisees usually pay for not only the supervision hour but also time devoted by the supervisor to listen to audio- or videotaped sessions. IPT therapists now exist throughout the world, which attests to the fact that geographic distance between IPT supervisor and supervisee can be overcome. Should psychotherapists who have not been formally supervised in IPT use it in clinical practice? Yes, but we believe that proficiency is built with supervision.

It is poignant and moving to provide psychotherapy to older people who are seriously depressed. One older woman remarked, "I'd rather have cancer than be depressed." Some older adults with depression have successfully dealt with a lifetime of challenges and now find it overwhelming to get out of bed in the morning. Given the significant functional impairment of major depression, some older adults with depression accomplish a remarkable amount despite the depression. As discussed in chapters 2, 3, and 4, the interpersonal dynamics of depression can be insidious and potentially destructive. Sometimes older people with depression are told by family and friends: "What do you have to be depressed about?" "If you try harder you'll get better." "Stop feeling sorry for yourself." "What's the problem? You've got a husband, money, and kids who call you." These messages convey blame to an individual who is suffering from an illness for which one symptom is self-blame. Average people often find it difficult to understand that major depression is a different animal than the intermittent dysphoria that is part and parcel of life. Understanding what it is like to live with depression can even be difficult for some mental health professionals. Mental health professionals who themselves have experienced major depression likely have a better appreciation of the often heroic struggles of persons with depression to get through each day. And deep gratification can come from lending a therapeutic hand to someone who is depressed and seeing that through the combined efforts of therapist and client, depression has lifted and the satisfactions life has to offer are once again enjoyed.

RESOURCES

GERONTOLOGY AND GEROPSYCHOLOGY
BIBLIOGRAPHIC RESOURCES

Birren, J. E., & Schroots, J. J. F. (Eds.). (2000). *A history of geropsychology in autobiography*. Washington, DC: American Psychological Association.

> In this book of narratives, prominent gerontologists and geropsychologists discuss personal and professional aspects of their careers in aging. The book will be helpful for those interested in understanding the evolution of contemporary geropsychology.

Cavanaugh, J. C., & Blanchard-Fields, F. (2002). *Adult development and aging* (4th ed.). Belmont, CA: Wadsworth/Thompson Learning.

> This undergraduate textbook provides a broad overview of major issues in gerontology with an emphasis on cognitive aging. The authors are well-known gerontology researchers and academics.

Duffy, M. (Ed.). (1999). *Handbook of counseling and psychotherapy with older adults*. New York: Wiley.

> This large edited volume is written by clinical and counseling geropsychologists. The handbook addresses issues in psychotherapy process with older adults; group and expressive therapy approaches; social and community interventions; and treatment approaches for selected problems.

Frazer, D. W., & Longsma, A. E. (1999). *The older adult psychotherapy treatment planner*. New York: Wiley.

> The volume is part of a larger series in which specific clinical problems, their assessment, and treatments are outlined. The book would be especially useful for those new to the delivery of psychological services to older adults.

Genevay, B., & Katz, R. S. (Eds.). (1990). *Countertransference and older adults*. Newbury Park, CA: Sage.

> This is one of the best books on countertransferential issues that may arise when delivering services to older people.

Hillman, J. L. (2000). *Clinical perspectives on elderly sexuality*. New York: Kluwer Academic/Plenum Publishers.

> This is an excellent summary of research on older adults' sexuality and treatment of late-life sexual problems.

Karel, M. J., Ogland-Hand, S., & Gatz, M. (with Jurgen Unutzer). (2002). *Assessing and treating late-life depression: A casebook and resource guide*. New York: Basic Books.

> This is our favorite book on late-life depression. It provides empirically grounded information on the assessment and treatment of depression in older adults. It is rich with clinical material that will be useful to practitioners.

Knight, B. G. (2004). *Psychotherapy with older adults* (3rd ed.). New York: Sage.

This classic text on psychotherapy with the aged was written by a prominent geropsychologist and researcher. It is highly recommended.

McIntosh, J. L., Santos, J. F., Hubbard, R. W., & Overholser, J. C. (1994). *Elder suicide: Research, theory, and treatment.* Washington, DC: American Psychological Association.

The volume is an excellent summary of research and clinical perspectives on late-life suicide.

Miller, M. D., & Reynolds, C. F. (2003). *Living longer depression free: A family guide to recognizing, treating, and preventing depression in later life.* Baltimore: Johns Hopkins University Press.

An excellent book for older adults with depression and their family members.

Molinari, V. (Ed.). (2000). *Professional psychology in long term care: A comprehensive guide.* New York: Hatherleigh Press.

For those delivering services to older adults in long-term care settings, this book is one of the best available. It is edited and written by geropsychologists who are well known in the field.

Moody, H. R. (2002). *Aging: Concepts and controversies* (4th ed.). Thousand Oaks, CA: Pine Forge Press.

This undergraduate textbook is organized around current ethical and policy issues related to aging. Those teaching gerontology will find that the book actively engages students in discussion.

Vierck, E., & Hodges, K. (2003). *Aging: Demographics, health, and health services.* Westport, CT: Greenwood Press.

This book makes facts on aging an intriguing topic.

Whitbourne, S. K. (Ed.). (2000). *Psychopathology in later adulthood.* New York: Wiley.

This edited volume provides readily accessible information on the most common clinical problems of older adults. Clinical material is woven throughout each chapter in a way that is helpful to clinicians.

Zarit, S. H., & Zarit, J. M. (1998). *Mental disorders in older adults: Fundamentals of assessment and treatment.* New York: Guilford Press.

For those seeking a research-supported and clinically useful overview of geropsychology, this is the best text. Steven Zarit is a highly regarded gerontologist who is best known for his research in late-life caregiving.

PROFESSIONAL RESOURCES IN GERONTOLOGY AND GEROPSYCHOLOGY

American Psychological Association's Division 12, Section II. http://www.geropsych.org

Section II, the Clinical Geropsychology section of Division 12 (Society of Clinical Psychology), is the primary professional home of those delivering psychological services to older adults. The Web site contains Section newsletters, directories of internship and postdoctoral training in geropsychology, reimbursement information, and information about membership.

American Psychological Association's Division 20 (Adult Development and Aging). http://www.apadiv20.phhp.ufl.edu

The Web site contains information about Division 20, a list of Division 20 members, resources for clinicians, educators, and students, upcoming conferences, and links to aging organizations and resources.

American Psychological Association's Office on Aging. http://www.apa.org/pi/aging/cona01.html

APA's Office on Aging works with the Association's Committee on Aging. The Web site provides access to a range of brochures, fact sheets, policy statements and guidelines, reports, and articles as well as recommended lists of journals, books, and videos. The Web site is an excellent resource for practicing geropsychologists.

The Department of Veterans Affairs. http://www.va.gov/oaa/AHE_default.asp

The VA has been a leader in the delivery of services to older veterans and in the training of psychologists and other health professionals. The VA Web site contains information on educational and training opportunities in VA centers throughout the country and links to VA jobs.

The Gerontological Society of America (GSA). http://www.geron.org

GSA is a large, interdisciplinary organization primarily devoted to the scientific study of aging. It has a mental health and aging interest group.

Psychologists in Long-Term Care (PLTC). http://www.wvu.edu/~pltc

PLTC is a group of psychologists who provide mental health services in long-term-care settings. The group has pioneered articulation of professional standards for delivery of psychological services in long-term care and is the primary professional home of psychologists with interests in this area.

IPT BIBLIOGRAPHIC RESOURCES

Markowitz, J. C. (1998). *Interpersonal psychotherapy for dysthymic disorder*. Washington, DC: American Psychiatric Press.

The book provides a clinically useful overview of relevant research on dysthymia as well as a manual for the IPT treatment of persons with the condition.

Weissman, M. M. (1995). *Mastering depression through interpersonal psychotherapy* and *Monitoring forms booklet*.

Available through the Psychological Corporation, Order Service Center, PO Box 839954, San Antonio, TX 78283-3954. These are educational materials developed for those being treated with IPT.

Weissman, M. M., Markowitz, J. C., & Klerman, G. L. (2000). *Comprehensive guide to interpersonal psychotherapy*. New York: Basic Books.

This is the definitive book on IPT; it contains the IPT manual, numerous clinical examples, and summaries of IPT research. For those interested in conducting IPT, it is a critical resource.

Wilfley, D. E., MacKenzie, K. R., Welch, R. R., Ayres, V. E., & Weissman, M. M. (2002). *Interpersonal psychotherapy for group*. New York: Basic Books.

Wilfley and colleagues have developed a group application of IPT. The book describes the use of group IPT in the treatment of depression and eating disorders. The volume is especially well written and clinically useful.

PROFESSIONAL RESOURCES IN IPT

International Society for Interpersonal Psychotherapy. http://www.interpersonalpsychotherapy.org

The Society is a professional and scientific organization with the mission of providing accurate information on the application of IPT. The Society's Web site contains a list of IPT-relevant publications, clinical applications of IPT, and training and events, as well as information on membership. In 2004 the organization had its first international meeting.

REFERENCES

Administration on Aging. (2001). *Older adults and mental health: Issues and opportunities*. Retrieved June 5, 2003, from http://www.aoa.gov/mh/report 2001/chapter1/ html

Agras, W. S., Walsh, T., Fairburn, C. G., Wilson, G. T., & Kraemer, H. C. (2000). A multicenter comparison of cognitive-behavioral and interpersonal psychotherapy for bulimia nervosa. *Archives of General Psychiatry, 57,* 459–466.

Alexopoulos, G., Meyers, B., Young, R., Campbell, S., Silbersweig, D., & Charlson, M. (1997). 'Vascular depression' hypothesis. *Archives of General Psychiatry, 54,* 915–922.

American Psychiatric Association. (1994). *Diagnostic and statistical manual of mental disorders* (4th ed.). Washington, DC: Author.

American Psychological Association. (2004). Guidelines for psychological practice with older adults. *American Psychologist, 59,* 236–260.

Aneshensel, C. S., Pearlin, L. I., Mullan, J. T., Zarit, S. H., & Whitlatch, C. J. (1995). *Profiles in caregiving: The unexpected career*. San Diego, CA: Academic Press.

APA Working Group on the Older Adult. (1998). What practitioners should know about working with older adults. *Professional Psychology: Research and Practice, 29,* 413–427.

Arbuckle, T. Y., Nohara-LeClair, M., & Pushkar, D. (2000). Effect of off-target verbosity on communication efficiency in a referential communication task. *Psychology & Aging, 15,* 65–77.

Arean, P. A., Perri, M. G., Nezu, A. M., Schein, R. L., Christopher, F., & Joseph, T. X. (1993). Comparative effectiveness of social problem-solving therapy and reminiscence therapy as treatment for depression in older adults. *Journal of Consulting and Clinical Psychology, 61,* 1003–1010.

Baldwin, R. C. (2000). Poor prognosis of depression in elderly people: Causes and actions. *Annals of Medicine, 32,* 252–256.

Beach, S. R. H., Sandeen, E. E., & O'Leary, D. K. (1990). *Depression in marriage*. New York: Guilford Press.

Beach, S. R., Schulz, R., Yee, J. L., & Jackson, S. (2000). Negative and positive health effects of caring for a disabled spouse: Longitudinal findings from the caregiver health effects study. *Psychology & Aging, 15,* 259–271.

Beck, A. T., Rush, A. J., Shaw, B. F., & Emery, G. (1979). *Cognitive therapy of depression*. New York: Guilford Press.

Binstock, R. H. (1985). The aged as scapegoat. In B. B. Hess & E. W. Markson (Eds.), *Growing old in America: New perspectives on old age* (3rd ed., pp. 489–506). New Brunswick, NJ: Transaction.

Binstock, R. H., & Quadagno, J. (2001). Aging and politics. In R. H. Binstock & L. K. George (Eds.), *Handbook of aging and the social sciences* (5th ed., pp. 333–351). San Diego, CA: Academic Press.

Blazer, D. G. (2003). Depression in late life: Review and commentary. *Journals of Gerontology: Medical Sciences, 58A*, 249–265.

Blazer, D. G. (2004). The psychiatric interview of older adults. In D. G. Blazer, D. C. Steffens, & E. W. Busse (Eds.), *Textbook of geriatric psychiatry* (3rd ed., pp. 165–177). Washington, DC: American Psychiatric Publishing.

Bleiberg, K. L., & Markowitz, J. C. (2005). A pilot study of interpersonal psychotherapy for posttraumatic stress disorder. *American Journal of Psychiatry, 162*, 181–183.

Bolton, P., Bass, J., Neugebauer, R., Verdeli, H., Clougherty, K. F., Wickramaratne, P. J., et al. (2003). A clinical trial of group interpersonal psychotherapy for depression in rural Uganda. *Journal of the American Medical Association, 289*, 3117–3124.

Bonanno, G. A., & Kaltman, S. (2001). The varieties of grief experience. *Clinical Psychology Review, 21*, 705–734.

Bookwala, J., & Schulz, R. (1996). Spousal similarity in subjective well-being: The cardiovascular health study. *Psychology and Aging, 11*, 582–590.

Bosworth, H. B., Hays, J. C., George, L. K., & Steffens, D. C. (2002). Psychosocial and clinical predictors of unipolar depression outcome in older adults. *International Journal of Geriatric Psychiatry, 17*, 238–246.

Bosworth, H. B., McQuoid, D. R., George, D. K., & Steffens, D. C. (2002). Time-to-remission from geriatric depression: Psychosocial and clinical factors. *American Journal of Geriatric Psychiatry, 10*, 551–559.

Brody, A. L., Saxena, S., Stoessel, P., Gillies, L. A., Fairbanks, L. A., Alborzian, S., et al. (2001). Regional brain metabolic changes in patients with major depression treated with either paroxetine or interpersonal therapy. *Archives of General Psychiatry, 58*, 631–640.

Brody, E. M. (1985). Parent care as a normative family stress. *The Gerontologist, 25*, 19–29.

Brokaw, T. (1999). *The greatest generation speaks.* New York: Random House.

Browne, G., Steiner, M., Roberts, J., Gafni, A., Byrne, C., Dunn, E., et al. (2002). Sertraline and/or interpersonal psychotherapy for patients with dysthymic disorder in primary care: 6-month comparison with longitudinal 2-year follow-up of effectiveness and costs. *Journal of Affective Disorders, 68*, 317–330.

Butler, R. (1963). The life review: An interpretation of reminiscence in the aged. *Psychiatry, 26*, 65–76.

Butler, R. (1975). *Why survive? Being old in America.* New York: HarperCollins.

Butzlaff, R. L., & Hooley, J. M. (1998). Expressed emotion and psychiatric relapse: A meta-analysis. *Archives of General Psychiatry, 55*, 547–552.

Caine, E. D., Lyness, J. M., & Conwell, Y. (1996). Diagnosis of late-life depression: Preliminary studies in primary care settings. *American Journal of Geriatric Psychiatry, 4*, S45–S50.

Carpenter, B., Ruckdeschel, K., Ruckdeschel, H., & Van Haitsma, K. (2002). R-E-M psychotherapy: A manualized approach for long-term care residents with depression and dementia. *Clinical Gerontologist, 25*, 25–49.

Carstensen, L. L., Gottman, J. M., & Levenson, R. W. (1995). Emotional behavior in long-term marriage. *Psychology and Aging, 10,* 140–149.

Chambless, D. L., Sanderson, W. C., Shoham, V., Johnson, S. B., Pope, K. S., Crits-Christoph, P., et al. (1996). An update on empirically validated therapies. *The Clinical Psychologist, 49,* 5–18.

Charney, D. S., Reynolds, C. F., Lewis, L., Lebowitz, B. D., Sunderland, T., Alexopoulos, G. S., et al. (2003). Depression and bipolar support alliance consensus statement on the unmet needs in diagnosis and treatment of mood disorders in late life. *Archives of General Psychiatry, 60,* 664–672.

Cole, M. G., & Bellavance, F. (1997). The prognosis of depression in old age. *American Journal of Geriatric Psychiatry, 5,* 4–14.

Congressional Budget Office. (1993, September). *Baby boomers in retirement: An early perspective* (CBO Publication No. 1993-343-277–814/96904). Washington, DC: U.S. Government Printing Office.

Coryell, W., Scheftner, W., Keller, M., Endicott, J., Maser, J., & Klerman, G. L. (1993). The enduring psychosocial consequences of mania and depression. *American Journal of Psychiatry, 150,* 720–727.

Cox, C. (1997). Findings from a statewide program of respite care: A comparison of service users, stoppers, and non-users. *The Gerontologist, 37,* 511–517.

Coyne, J. C. (1976). Depression and the response of others. *Journal of Abnormal Psychology, 85,* 186–193.

Crowley, B. J., Hayslip, B., & Hobdy, J. (2003). Psychological hardiness and adjustment to life events in adulthood. *Journal of Adult Development, 10,* 237–248.

Crown, W. (2001). Economic status of the elderly. In R. W. Binstock & L. K. George (Eds.), *Handbook of aging and the social sciences* (5th ed., pp. 352–368). San Diego, CA: Academic Press.

DiMascio, A., Weissman, M. M., Prusoff, B. A., Neu, C., Zwilling, M., & Klerman, G. L. (1979). Differential symptom reduction by drugs and psychotherapy in acute depression. *Archives of General Psychiatry, 36,* 1450–1456.

Donnelly, J. M., Kornblith, A. B., Fleishman, S., Zuckerman, E., Raptis, G., Hudis, C. A., et al. (2000). A pilot study of interpersonal psychotherapy by telephone with cancer patients and their partners. *Psycho-Oncology, 9,* 44–56.

Elkin, I., Shea, M. T., Watkins, J. T., Imber, S. D., Sotsky, S. M., Collins, J. F., et al. (1989). National Institute of Mental Health treatment of depression collaborative research program: General effectiveness of treatments. *Archives of General Psychiatry, 46,* 971–982.

Erikson, E. H. (1980). *Identity and the life cycle.* New York: Norton.

Estes, C., & Binney, E. A. (1989). The biomedicalization of aging: Dangers and dilemmas. *The Gerontologist, 29,* 587–596.

Fairburn, C. G., Jones, R., Peveler, R. C., Carr, S. J., Solomon, R. A., O'Connor, M. E., et al. (1991). Three psychological treatments for bulimia nervosa: A comparative trial. *Archives of General Psychiatry, 48,* 463–469.

Federal Interagency Forum on Aging-Related Statistics. (2000, August). *Older Americans 2000: Key indicators of well-being.* Washington, DC: U.S. Government Printing Office.

Federal Interagency Forum on Aging-Related Statistics. (2004, November). *Older Americans 2004: Key indicators of well-being.* Washington, DC: U.S. Government Printing Office.

Foley, S. H., Rounsaville, B. J., Weissman, M. M., Sholomskas, D., & Chevron, E. (1989). Individual versus conjoint interpersonal psychotherapy for depressed patients with marital disputes. *International Journal of Family Psychiatry, 10,* 29–42.

Folstein, M. F., Folstein, S. E., & McHugh, P. R. (1975). "Mini-Mental State." A practical method for grading the cognitive state of patients for the clinician. *Journal of Psychiatric Research, 12,* 189–198.

Frank, E. (1991). Interpersonal psychotherapy as a maintenance treatment for patients with recurrent depression. *Psychotherapy, 28,* 259–266.

Frank, E., Hlastala, S., Ritenour, A., Houck, P., Tu, X. M., Monk, T. H., et al. (1997). Inducing lifestyle regularity in recovering bipolar disorder patients: Results from the maintenance therapies in bipolar disorder protocol. *Biological Psychiatry, 41,* 1165–1173.

Frank, E., Kupfer, D. J., Perel, J. M., Cornes, C., Jarrett, D. B., Mallinger, A. G., et al. (1990). Three-year outcomes for maintenance therapies in recurrent depression. *Archives of General Psychiatry, 47,* 1093–1099.

Frank, E., Kupfer, D. J., Wagner, E. F., McEachran, A. B., & Cornes, C. (1991). Efficacy of interpersonal psychotherapy as a maintenance treatment of recurrent depression: Contributing factors. *Archives of General Psychiatry, 48,* 1053–1059.

Frank, E., & Spanier, C. (1995). Interpersonal psychotherapy for depression: Overview, clinical efficacy, and future directions. *Clinical Psychology: Science and Practice, 2,* 349–369.

Friedmann, M. S., McDermut, W. H., Solomon, D. A., Ryan, C. E., Keitner, G. I., & Miller, I. W. (1997). Family functioning and mental illness: A comparison of psychiatric and nonclinical families. *Family Process, 36,* 357–367.

Fry, P. S. (1983). Structured and unstructured reminiscence training and depression among the elderly. *Clinical Gerontologist, 1,* 15–37.

Gallagher-Thompson, D., Hanley-Peterson, P., & Thompson, L. W. (1990). Maintenance of gains versus relapse following brief psychotherapy for depression. *Journal of Consulting and Clinical Psychology, 58,* 371–374.

Gallagher-Thompson, D., & Steffen, A. (1994). Comparative effects of cognitive/behavioral and brief psychodynamic psychotherapies for depressed family caregivers. *Journal of Counseling and Clinical Psychology, 62,* 543–549.

Gallagher-Thompson, D., & Thompson, L. W. (1996). Bereavement and adjustment disorders. In E. W. Busse & D. G. Blazer (Eds.), *Textbook of geriatric psychiatry* (2nd ed., pp. 313–328). Washington, DC: American Psychiatric Press.

Gatz, M., & Finkel, S. I. (1995). Education and training of mental health service providers. In M. Gatz (Ed.), *Emerging issues in mental health and aging* (pp. 282–302). Washington, DC: American Psychological Association.

Gatz, M., Fiske, A., Fox, L. S., Kaskie, B., Kasl-Godley, J. E., McCallum, T. J., & Wetherell, J. L. (1999). Empirically validated psychological treatment for older adults. *Journal of Mental Health and Aging, 4,* 9–46.

Genevay, B., & Katz, R. S. (Eds.). (1990). *Countertransference and older adults.* Newbury Park, CA: Sage.

George, L. K. (1994). Social factors and depression in late life. In L. S. Schneider, C. F. Reynolds, B. D. Lebowitz, & A. J. Friedhoff (Eds.), *Diagnosis and treatment of depression in late life* (pp. 131–154). Washington, DC: American Psychiatric Press.

George, L. K. (2004). Social and economic factors related to psychiatric disorders in late life. In D. G. Blazer, D. C. Steffens, & E. W. Busse (Eds.), *Textbook of geriatric psychiatry* (3rd ed., pp. 139–161). Washington, DC: American Psychiatric Publishing.

Georgotas, A., McCue, R. E., Hapworth, W., Friedman, E., Kim, O. M., Welkowitz, J., et al. (1986). Comparative efficacy and safety of MAOI vs. TCAs in treating depression in the elderly. *Biological Psychiatry, 21,* 1155–1166.

Goodman, C. R., & Shippy, R. A. (2002). Is it contagious? Affect similarity among spouses. *Aging & Mental Health, 6,* 266–274.

Gotlib, I. H., & Beach, S. R. H. (1995). A marital/family discord model of depression: Implications for therapeutic intervention. In N. S. Jacobson & A. S. Gurman (Eds.), *Handbook of couple therapy* (pp. 411–436). New York: Guilford Press.

Gurland, B. J., Dean, L. L., & Cross, P. S. (1983). The effects of depression on individual social functioning in the elderly. In L. D. Breslau & M. R. Haug (Eds.), *Depression and aging: Causes, care, and consequences* (pp. 256–265). New York: Springer.

Haight, B. K. (1988). The therapeutic role of a structured life review process in homebound elderly subjects. *Journal of Gerontology: Psychological Sciences, 43,* P40–P44.

Haight, B. K. (1992). Long-term effects of a structured life review process. *Journals of Gerontology: Psychological Sciences, 47,* P312–P315.

Hamilton, M. (1960). A rating scale for depression. *Journal of Neurology and Neurosurgical Psychiatry, 23,* 56–62.

Hanson, R. O., & Hayslip, B. (2000). Widowhood in later life. In J. H. Harvey & E. D. Miller (Eds.), *Loss and trauma: General and close relationship perspectives* (pp. 345–357). Philadelphia: Brunner-Routledge.

Herzog, A. R., & Markus, H. R. (1999). The self concept in life span and aging research. In V. L. Bengtson & K. W. Schaie (Eds.), *Handbook of theories of aging* (pp. 227–252). New York: Springer.

Higgins, E. S. (1994). A review of unrecognized mental illness in primary care: Prevalence, natural history, and efforts to change the course. *Archives of Family Medicine, 3,* 908–917.

Hinrichsen, G. A. (1992). Recovery and relapse from major depressive disorder in the elderly. *American Journal of Psychiatry, 149*, 1575–1579.

Hinrichsen, G. A. (1997). Interpersonal psychotherapy for depressed older adults. *Journal of Geriatric Psychiatry, 30*, 239–257.

Hinrichsen, G. A. (1999). Treating older adults with interpersonal psychotherapy of depression. *Journal of Clinical Psychology: In Session: Psychotherapy in Practice, 55*, 949–960.

Hinrichsen, G. A. (2000). Knowledge of and interest in geropsychology among psychology trainees. *Professional Psychology: Research and Practice, 31*, 442–445.

Hinrichsen, G. A. (2004, June). *Training in and application of IPT in a geriatric outpatient setting.* Paper presented at the First International Conference on Interpersonal Psychotherapy, Pittsburgh, PA.

Hinrichsen, G. A., Adelstein, L., & McMeniman, M. (2004). Expressed emotion in family members of depressed older adults. *Aging and Mental Health: An International Journal, 8*, 343–351.

Hinrichsen, G. A., & Emery, E. E. (2005). Interpersonal factors and late-life depression. *Clinical Psychology: Science and Practice, 12*, 264–275.

Hinrichsen, G. A., & Hernandez, N. A. (1993). Factors associated with recovery from and relapse into major depressive disorder in the elderly. *American Journal of Psychiatry, 150*, 1820–1825.

Hinrichsen, G. A., Hernandez, N. A., & Pollack, S. (1992). Difficulties and rewards in family care of the depressed older adult. *Gerontologist, 32*, 486–492.

Hinrichsen, G. A., & Pollack, S. (1997). Expressed emotion and the course of late-life depression. *Journal of Abnormal Psychology, 106*, 336–340.

Hirschfeld, R. M. A., Montgomery, S. A., Keller, M. B., Kasper, S., Schatzberg, A. F., Moller, H., et al. (2000). Social functioning in depression: A review. *Journal of Clinical Psychiatry, 61*, 268–275.

Hooker, K. (1999). Possible selves in adulthood: Incorporating teleonomic relevance into studies of the self. In T. M. Hess & F. Blanchard-Fields (Eds.), *Social cognition and aging* (pp. 97–122). San Diego, CA: Academic Press.

Hooley, J. M., Orley, J., & Teasdale, D. J. (1986). Levels of expressed emotion and relapse in depressed patients. *British Journal of Psychiatry, 148*, 642–647.

Hooyman, N., & Kiyak, H. A. (1999). *Social gerontology: A multidisciplinary perspective* (5th ed.). Boston: Allyn & Bacon.

Horn, J. L. (1982). The aging of human abilities. In B. B. Wolman (Ed.), *Handbook of developmental psychology* (pp. 847–870). Englewood Cliffs, NJ: Prentice Hall.

Horvath, P. (1988). Placebos and common factors in two decades of psychotherapy research. *Psychological Bulletin, 104*, 214–225.

Hoyl, M. T., Alessi, C. A., Harker, J. O., Josephson, K. R., Pietruszka, F. M., Koelfgen, M., et al. (1999). Development and testing of a five-item version of the Geriatric Depression Scale. *Journal of the American Geriatrics Society, 47*, 873–878.

Huyck, M. H. (1990). Gender differences in aging. In J. E. Birren & K. W. Schaie (Eds.), *Handbook of the psychology of aging* (3rd ed., pp. 124–132). San Diego, CA: Academic Press.

Jeste, D. V., Alexopoulos, G. S., Bartels, S. J., Cummings, J. L., Gallo, J. J., Gottlieb, G. L., et al. (1999). Consensus statement on the upcoming crisis in geriatric mental health. *Archives of General Psychiatry, 56,* 848–853.

Joiner, T. E. (2000). Depression's vicious scree: Self-propagating and erosive processes in depression chronicity. *Clinical Psychology: Science and Practice, 7,* 203–218.

Judd, L. L., & Akiskal, H. S. (2000). Delineating the longitudinal structure of depressive illness: Beyond clinical subtypes and duration thresholds. *Pharmacopsychiatry, 33,* 3–7.

Judd, L. L., Akiskal, H. G., Zeller, P. J., Paulus, M., Leon, A. C., Maser, J. D., et al. (2000). Psychosocial disability during the long-term course of unipolar major depressive disorder. *Archives of General Psychiatry, 57,* 375–380.

Karel, M. J. (1997). Aging and depression: Vulnerability and stress across adulthood. *Clinical Psychology Review, 17,* 847–879.

Karel, M. J., & Hinrichsen, G. (2000). Treatment of depression in late life: Psychotherapeutic interventions. *Clinical Psychology Review, 20,* 707–729.

Karel, M. J., Ogland-Hand, S., & Gatz, M. (with Unutzer, J). (2002). *Assessing and treating late-life depression: A casebook and resource guide.* New York: Basic Books.

Karlin, B. E., & Duffy, M. (2004). Geriatric mental health policy: Impact on service delivery and directions for effecting change. *Professional Psychology: Research & Practice, 35,* 509–519.

Kawachi, I., & Berkman, L. F. (2001). Social ties and mental health. *Journal of Urban Health: Bulletin of the New York Academy of Medicine, 78,* 458–467.

Keitner, G. I., & Miller, I. W. (1990). Family functioning and major depression: An overview. *American Journal of Psychiatry, 147,* 1128–1137.

Keller, M. B., Klerman, G. L., Lavori, P. W., Fawcett, J. A., Coryell, W., & Endicott, J. (1982). Treatment received by depressed patients. *Journal of the American Medical Association, 248,* 1848–1855.

Keller, M. B., Lavori, P. W., & Mueller, T. I. (1992). Time to recovery, chronicity, and levels of psychopathology in major depression: A five-year prospective follow-up of 431 subjects. *Archives of General Psychiatry, 49,* 809–816.

Keller, M. B., & Shapiro, R. W. (1981). Major depressive disorder: Initial results from a one-year prospective naturalistic follow-up study. *Journal of Nervous and Mental Disease, 169,* 761–767.

Keller, M. B., & Shapiro, R. W. (1982). "Double depression": Superimposition of acute depressive episodes on chronic depressive disorders. *American Journal of Psychiatry, 139,* 438–442.

Kimmel, D. C. (2002). Aging and sexual orientation. In J. Oldham (Series Ed.), M. Riba (Series Ed.), B. E. Jones (Vol. Ed.), & M. J. Hill (Vol. Ed.), *Review of Psychiatry: Vol. 21. Mental health issues in lesbian, gay, bisexual and transgender communities* (pp. 17–36). Washington, DC: American Psychiatric Publishing.

King, D. A., Shields, C. G., & Wynne, L. C. (2000). Intervention and consultation with families of older adults. In B. J. Sadock & V. A. Sadock (Eds.), *The compre-*

hensive textbook of psychiatry (7th ed., pp. 3122–3127). Philadelphia: Lippincott Williams & Wilkins.

Kingson, E. R., & Schulz, J. H. (1997). *Social security in the 21st century.* New York: Oxford University Press.

Klein, D. F., & Ross, D. C. (1993). Reanalysis of the National Institute of Mental Health Treatment of Depression Collaborative Research Program general effectiveness report. *Neuropsychopharmacology, 8,* 241–251.

Klerman, G. L., Budman, S., Berwick, D., Weissman, M. M., Damico-White, J., Demby, A., & Feldstein, M. (1987). Efficacy of a brief psychosocial intervention for symptoms of stress and distress among patients in primary care. *Medical Care, 25,* 1078–1088.

Klerman, G. L., DiMascio, A., Weissman, M., Prusoff, B., & Paykel, E. (1974). Treatment of depression by drugs and psychotherapy. *American Journal of Psychiatry, 131,* 186–191.

Klerman, G. L., & Weissmann, M. M. (1989). Increasing rates of depression. *Journal of the American Medical Association, 261,* 2229–2235.

Klerman, G. L., Weissman, M. M., Rounsaville, B. J., & Chevron, E. S. (1984). *Interpersonal psychotherapy of depression.* Northvale, NJ: Jason Aronson.

Knight, B. (2004). *Psychotherapy with older adults* (3rd ed.). Thousand Oaks, CA: Sage.

Kupfer, D. J., Frank, E., Perel, J. M., Cornes, C., & Mallinger, V. J. (1992). Five-year outcome for maintenance therapies in recurrent depression. *Archives of General Psychiatry, 49,* 769–773.

Lawton, M. P., & Nahemow, L. (1973). Ecology and the aging process. In C. Eisdorfer & M. P. Lawton (Eds.), *The psychology of adult development and aging* (pp. 619–674). Washington, DC: American Psychological Association.

Lazarus, R. S., & Folkman, S. (1984). *Stress, appraisal, and coping.* New York: Springer.

Lenze, E. J., Dew, M. A., Mazumdar, S., Begley, A. E., Cornes, C., Miller, M. D., et al. (2002). Combined pharmacotherapy and psychotherapy as maintenance treatment for late-life depression: Effects on social adjustment. *American Journal of Psychiatry, 159,* 466–468.

Lenze, E. J., Rogers, J. C., Martire, L. M., Mulsant, B. H., Rollman, B. L., Dew, M. A., et al. (2001). The association of late-life depression and anxiety with physical disability: A review of the literature and prospectus for future research. *American Journal of Geriatric Psychiatry, 9,* 113–134.

Levant, R. F. (2004). The empirically validated treatments movement: A practitioner/educator perspective. *Clinical Psychology: Science and Practice, 11,* 219–224.

Levinson, D. J. (with Darrow, C. N., Klein, E. B., Levinson, M. H., & McKee, B.). (1978). *The seasons of a man's life.* New York: Knopf.

Levinson, D. J. (1986). A conception of adult development. *American Psychologist, 41,* 3–13.

Levy, B. R., & Banaji, M. R. (2002). Implicit ageism. In T. D. Nelson (Ed.), *Ageism: Stereotyping and prejudice against older persons* (pp. 49–75). Cambridge, MA: MIT Press.

Lipsitz, J. F., Markowitz, J. C., Cherry, S., & Fryer, A. J. (1999). Open trial of inter-personal psychotherapy for social phobia. *American Journal of Psychiatry, 156,* 1814–1816.

Liptzin, B., Grob, M. C., & Eisen, S. V. (1988). Family burden of demented and depressed elderly psychiatric inpatients. *Gerontologist, 28,* 397–401.

Lovett, S., & Gallagher, D. (1988). Psychoeducational interventions for family caregivers: Preliminary efficacy data. *Behavior Therapy, 19,* 321–330.

Maddox, G. L. (2001). Housing and living arrangements: A transactional perspec-tive. In R. H. Binstock & L. K. George (Eds.), *Handbook of aging and the social sciences* (5th ed., pp. 426–443). San Diego, CA: Academic Press.

Markowitz, J. C. (1998). *Interpersonal psychotherapy for dysthymic disorder.* Washing-ton, DC: American Psychiatric Press.

Markowitz, J. C., Kocsis, J. H., Fishman, B., Spielman, L. A., Jacobsberg, L. B., Frances, A. J., et al. (1999). Treatment of HIV-positive patients with depressive symp-toms. *Archives of General Psychiatry, 55,* 452–457.

Markus, H., & Nurius, P. (1986). Possible selves. *American Psychologist, 41,* 954–989.

Mazure, C. M. (1998). Life stressors as risk factors in depression. *Clinical Psychology: Science and Practice, 5,* 291–313.

McAdams, D. P. (1995). What do we know when we know a person? *Journal of Personality, 63,* 365–396.

McIntosh, J. L., Santos, J. F., Hubbard, R. W., & Overholser, J. C. (1994). *Elder suicide: Research, theory, and treatment.* Washington, DC: American Psychologi-cal Association.

Mello, M. F., Mari, J. J., Bacaltchuk, J., Verdeli, H., & Neugebauer, R. (2005). A systematic review of research findings on the efficacy of interpersonal therapy for depressive disorders. *European Archives of Psychiatry and Clinical Neuroscience, 255,* 75–82.

Mello, M. F., Myczowisk, L. M., & Menezes, P. R. (2001). A randomized controlled trial comparing moclobemide and moclobemide plus interpersonal psychotherapy in the treatment of dysthymic disorder. *Journal of Psychotherapy Practice & Re-search, 10,* 117–123.

Miller, M. D. (2004, March). *Using IPT in depressed elders with cognitive dysfunction.* Paper presented at the annual meeting of the American Association of Geriat-ric Psychiatry, Baltimore, MD.

Miller, M. D., Frank, E., Cornes, C., Houck, P. R., & Reynolds, C. F., III. (2003). The value of maintenance interpersonal psychotherapy (IPT) in older adults with different IPT foci. *American Journal of Geriatric Psychiatry, 11,* 97–102.

Miller, M. D., & Silberman, R. L. (1996). Using interpersonal psychotherapy with depressed elders. In S. H. Zarit & B. G. Knight (Eds.), *A guide to psychotherapy and aging* (pp. 83–99). Washington, DC: American Psychological Association.

Miller, L., & Weissman, M. (2002). Interpersonal psychotherapy delivered over the telephone to recurrent depressives. A pilot study. *Depression & Anxiety, 16,* 114–117.

Molinari, V. (Ed.). (2000). *Professional psychology in long term care: A comprehensive guide*. New York: Hatherleigh Press.

Moody, H. R. (1998). *Aging: Concepts and controversies* (2nd ed.). Thousand Oaks, CA: Pine Forge Press.

Moss, M. S., Moss., S. Z., & Hansson, R. O. (2001). Bereavement and old age. In M. S. Stroebe, R. O. Hansson, W. Stroebe, & H. Schut (Eds.), *Handbook of bereavement research: Consequences, coping and care* (pp. 241–260). Washington, DC: American Psychological Association.

Mossey, J. M., Knott, K. A., Higgins, M., & Talerico, K. (1996). Effectiveness of a psychosocial intervention, interpersonal counseling, for subdysthymic depression in medically ill elderly. *Journal of Gerontology: Medical Sciences, 51A,* M172–M178.

Mufson, L., Gallagher, T., Dorta, K. P., & Young, J. F. (2004). A group adaptation of interpersonal psychotherapy for depressed adolescents. *American Journal of Psychotherapy, 58,* 220–237.

Mufson, L., Pollack Dorta, K., Moreau, D., & Weissman, M. M. (2004). *Interpersonal therapy for depressed adolescents* (2nd ed.). New York: Guilford Press.

Mulsant, B. H., & Pollack, B. G. (2004). Psychopharmacology. In D. G. Blazer, D. C. Steffens, & E. W. Busse (Eds.), *Textbook of geriatric psychiatry* (pp. 387–411). Washington, DC: American Psychiatric Publishing.

Murray, C. J. L., & Lopez, A. D. (1996). *The global burden of disease: A comprehensive assessment of mortality and disability from diseases, injuries, and risk factors in 1990 and projected to 2020*. Cambridge, MA: Harvard University Press.

National Institutes of Health. (1991). *Diagnosis and treatment of depression in late life* (Vol. 9, No. 3). Bethesda, MD: National Library of Medicine.

Neugarten, B. (1982). *Age or need? Public policies for older people*. Beverly Hills, CA: Sage.

Neugarten, B. L., & Neugarten, D. A. (1986). Changing meaning of age in the aging society. In A. Pifer & L. Bronte (Eds.), *Our aging society: Paradox and promise*. New York: Norton.

Newsom, J. T., & Schulz, R. (1998). Caregiving from the recipient's perspective: Negative reactions to being helped. *Health Psychology, 17,* 172–181.

O'Hara, M. W., Stuart, S., Gorman, L. L., & Wenzel, A. (2000). Efficacy of interpersonal psychotherapy for postpartum depression. *Archives of General Psychiatry, 57,* 1039–1045.

Palmore, E. (2001). The ageism survey: First findings. *The Gerontologist, 41,* 572–575.

Piaget, J. (1980). *Les formes et les mentaires de la dialectique*. Paris: Gallimard.

Pruchno, R. (1999). Raising grandchildren: The experiences of Black and White grandmothers. *The Gerontologist, 39,* 209–221.

Qualls, S. H. (1996). Family therapy with aging families. In S. H. Zarit & B. G. Knight (Eds.), *A guide to psychotherapy and aging* (pp. 121–137). Washington, DC: American Psychological Association.

Qualls, S. H., Segal, D., Norman, S., Niederehe, G., & Gallagher-Thompson, D. (2002). Psychologists in practice with older adults: Current patterns, sources of training, and need for continuing education. *Professional Psychology: Research and Practice, 33,* 435–442.

Raskind, M. A., Bonner, L. T., & Peskind, E. R. (2004). Cognitive disorders. In D. G. Blazer, D. C. Steffens, & E. W. Busse (Eds.), *Textbook of geriatric psychiatry* (pp. 207–229). Washington, DC: American Psychiatric Publishing.

Rattenbury, C., & Stones, M. J. (1989). A controlled evaluation of reminiscence and current topics discussion groups in a nursing home context. *Gerontologist, 29,* 768–771.

Reichman, W. E., & Katz, P. R. (Eds.). (1996). *Psychiatric care in the nursing home.* New York: Oxford University Press.

Reynolds, C. F., Alexopoulos, G. S., Katz, I. R., & Lebowitz, B. D. (2001). Chronic depression in the elderly. *Drugs and Aging, 18,* 507–514.

Reynolds, C. F., III, Frank, E., Perel, J. M., Imber, S. D., Cornes, C., Miller, M. D., et al. (1999). Nortriptyline and interpersonal psychotherapy as maintenance therapies for recurrent major depression: A randomized controlled trial in patients older than 59 years. *Journal of the American Medical Association, 281,* 39–45.

Reynolds, C. F., III, Kupfer, D. J., Thase, M. E., Perel, J. M., Mazumdar, S., & Houck, P. R. (1996). Treatment outcome in recurrent major depression: A posthoc comparison of elderly ("young old") and midlife patient. *American Journal of Psychiatry, 153,* 1288–1292.

Robins, L. N., & Regier, D. A. (Eds.). (1991). *Psychiatric disorders in America: The epidemiologic catchment area study.* New York: The Free Press.

Rose, J. M., & DelMaestro, S. G. (1990). Separation-individuation conflict as a model for understanding distressed caregivers: Psychodynamic and cognitive case studies. *The Gerontologist, 30,* 693–697.

Rosow, I. (1967). *Social integration of the aged.* New York: Free Press.

Rosowsky, E., Abrams, R. C., & Zweig, R. A. (Eds.). (1999). *Personality disorders in older adults: Emerging issues in diagnosis and treatment.* Mahwah, NJ: Erlbaum.

Rothblum, E. D., Sholomskas, A. J., Berry, C., & Prusoff, B. A. (1982). Issues in clinical trials with the depressed elderly. *Journal of the American Geriatrics Society, 30,* 694–699.

Rounsaville, B. J., Glazer, W., Wilber, C. H, Weissman, M. M., & Kleber, H. D. (1983). Short-term interpersonal psychotherapy in methadone-maintained opiate addicts. *Archives of General Psychiatry, 40,* 629–636.

Rubinstein, R. L. (1987). Never married elderly as a social type: Re-evaluating some images. *Gerontologist, 27,* 103–113.

Rubinstein, R. L., Alexander, B. B., Goodman, M., & Luborsky, M. (1991). Key relationships of never married, childless older women: A cultural analysis. *Journals of Gerontology, 46,* S270–S277.

Sackheim, H. A. (1994). Use of electroconvulsive therapy in late life depression. In L. S. Schneider, C. F. Reynolds, B. D. Lebowitz, & A. J. Friedhoff (Eds.), *Diag-*

nosis and treatment of depression in late life (pp. 259–277). Washington, DC: American Psychiatric Association Press.

Schaie, K. W. (1994). The course of adult intellectual development. *American Psychologist, 49,* 304–313.

Schulberg, H. C., Block, M. R., Madonia, M. J., Scott, P., Rodriguez, E., Imber, S. D., et al. (1996). Treating major depression in primary care practice. *Archives of General Psychiatry, 53,* 913–919.

Schulz, R., O'Brien, A. T., Bookwala, J., & Fleissner, K. (1995). Psychiatric and physical morbidity effects of dementia caregiving: Prevalence, correlates, and causes. *Gerontologist, 35,* 771–791.

Schulz, R., Visintainer, P., & Williamson, G. M. (1990). Psychiatric and physical morbidity effects of caregiving. *Journals of Gerontology: Psychological Sciences, 45,* 181–191.

Schut, H. A., Stroebe, M. S., de Keijser, J., & van den Bout, J. (1997). Intervention for the bereaved: Gender differences in the efficacy of two counselling programmes. *British Journal of Clinical Psychology, 36,* 63–72.

Scogin, F., Jamison, C., & Davis, N. (1990). Two-year follow-up of bibliotherapy for depression in older adults. *Journal of Consulting and Clinical Psychology, 58,* 665–667.

Scogin, F., Jamison, C., & Gochneaur, K. (1989). Comparative efficacy of cognitive and behavioral bibliotherapy for mildly and moderately depressed older adults. *Journal of Consulting and Clinical Psychology, 57,* 403–407.

Scogin, F., & McElreath, I. (1994). Efficacy of psychosocial treatments for geriatric depression: A quantitative review. *Journal of Consulting and Clinical Psychology, 57,* 403–407.

Selye, H. (1956). *The stress of life.* New York: McGraw-Hill.

Shanas, E. (1979). Social myth as hypothesis: The case of the family relations of old people. *The Gerontologist, 19,* 3–9.

Sheehy, G. (1977). *Passages: Predictable crises of adult life.* New York: Dutton.

Sheikh, J. I., & Yesavage, J. A. (1986). Geriatric Depression Scale (GDS): Recent evidence and development of a shorter version. *Clinical Gerontologist, 5,* 165–173.

Sholomskas, A. J., Chevron, E. S., Prusoff, B. A., & Berry, C. (1983). Short-term interpersonal therapy (IPT) with the depressed elderly: Case reports and discussion. *American Journal of Psychotherapy, 37,* 552–566.

Sloane, R. B., Staples, F. R., & Schneider, L. S. (1985). Interpersonal psychotherapy versus nortriptyline for depression in the elderly. In G. Burrows, T. R. Norman, & L. Dennerstein (Eds.), *Clinical and pharmacological studies in psychiatric disorders* (pp. 344–346). London: John Libbey.

Spinelli, M. G. (1997). Interpersonal psychotherapy for depressed pregnant HIV-positive women: A pilot study. *American Journal of Psychiatry, 154,* 1028–1030.

Spinelli, M. G., & Endicott, J. (2003). Controlled clinical trial of interpersonal psychotherapy versus parenting education program for depressed pregnant women. *American Journal of Psychiatry, 160,* 555–562.

Steuer, J. L., Mintz, J., Hammen, C. L., Hill, M. A., Jarvik, L. F., McCarley, T., et al. (1984). Cognitive-behavioral and psychodynamic group psychotherapy in treatment of geriatric depression. *Journal of Consulting and Clinical Psychology, 52,* 180–189.

Stuart, S., & O'Hara, M. W. (1995). Interpersonal psychotherapy for postpartum depression. *Journal of Psychotherapy Practice and Research, 4,* 18–29.

Sullivan, H. S. (1953). *The interpersonal theory of psychiatry.* New York: Norton.

Teng, E. L., & Chui, H. C. (1987). The Modified Mini-Mental State (3MS) Examination. *Journal of Clinical Psychiatry, 48,* 314–318.

Teri, L., Logsdon, R. G., Uomoto, J., & McCurry, S. M. (1997). Behavioral treatment of depression in dementia patients: A controlled clinical trial. *Journals of Gerontology: Psychological Sciences, 52B,* P159–P166.

Thompson, L. W., Gallagher, D., & Breckenridge, J. S. (1987). Comparative effectiveness of psychotherapies for depressed elders. *Journal of Consulting and Clinical Psychology, 55,* 385–390.

Tower, R. B., & Kasl, S. V. (1995). Depressive symptoms across older spouses and the moderating effect of marital closeness. *Psychology and Aging, 10,* 625–638.

Tower, R. B., & Kasl, S. V. (1996). Depressive symptoms across older spouses: Longitudinal influences. *Psychology and Aging, 11,* 683–697.

Unutzer, J., Katon, W., Callahan, C. M., Williams, J. W., Hunkeler, E., Harpole, L., et al. (2002). Collaborative care management of late-life depression in the primary care setting. *Journal of the American Medical Association, 288,* 2836–2845.

Verdeli, H., Clougherty, K. F., Bolton, P., Speelman, L., Ndogoni, L., Bass, J., et al. (2003). Adapting group interpersonal psychotherapy for a developing country: Experience in rural Uganda. *World Psychiatry, 2,* 114–120.

Vierck, E., & Hodges, K. (2003). *Aging: Demographics, health, and health services.* Westport, CT: Greenwood Press.

Wei, W., Sambamoorthi, U., Olfson, M., Walkup, J. T., & Crystal, S. (2005). Use of psychotherapy for depression in older adults. *American Journal of Psychiatry, 162,* 711–717.

Weiss, R. S. (1974). The provisions of social relationships. In Z. Rubin (Ed.), *Doing unto others* (pp. 17–26). Englewood Cliffs, NJ: Prentice-Hall.

Weissman, M. M. (1995). *Mastering depression through interpersonal psychotherapy* and *Monitoring forms booklet.* Available through the Psychological Corporation, Order Service Center, PO Box 839954, San Antonio, TX 78283–3954.

Weissman, M. M., Bruce, M. L., Leaf, P. L., Florio, L. P., & Holzer, C., III (1991). Affective disorders. In L. N. Robins & D. A. Regier (Eds.), *Psychiatric disorders in America: The epidemiologic catchment area study* (pp. 53–80). New York: The Free Press.

Weissman, M. M., Klerman, G. L., Prusoff, B. A., Sholomskas, D., & Padian, N. (1981). Depressed outpatients: Results one year after treatment with drugs and/or interpersonal psychotherapy. *Archives of General Psychiatry, 38,* 51–55.

Weissman, M. M., Markowitz, J. C., & Klerman, G. L. (2000). *Comprehensive guide to interpersonal psychotherapy.* New York: Basic Books.

Weissman, M. M., & Paykel, E. (1974). *The depressed woman*. Chicago: University of Chicago Press.

Weissman, M. M., Prusoff, B. A., DiMascio, A., Neu, C., Goklaney, M., & Klerman, G. L. (1979). The efficacy of drugs and psychotherapy in the treatment of acute depressive episodes. *American Journal of Psychiatry, 134,* 555–558.

Wells, K. B., Stewart, A., Hays, R. D., Burnam, A., Rogers, W., Daniels, M., et al. (1989). The functioning and well-being of depressed patients: Results from the Medical Outcomes Study. *Journal of the American Medical Association, 262,* 914–919.

Whitbourne, S. K. (1987). Personality development in adulthood and old age. Relationships among identity style, health, and well being. In K. W. Schaie (Ed.), *Annual review of gerontology and geriatrics: Vol. 7. Experimental and applied psychology* (pp. 189–216). New York: Springer.

Whitbourne, S. K. (1999). Physical changes. In J. C. Cavanaugh & S. K. Whitbourne (Eds.), *Gerontology: Interdisciplinary perspectives* (pp. 91–122). New York: Oxford University Press.

Wickramaratne, P. J., Weissman, M. M., Leaf, P. J., & Holford, T. R. (1989). Age, period and cohort effects on the risk of major depression: Results from five United States communities. *Journal of Clinical Epidemiology, 42,* 333–343.

Wilfley, D. E., Agras, W. S., Telch, C. F., Rossiter, E. M., Schneider, J. A., Cole, A. G., et al. (1993). Group cognitive-behavior therapy and group interpersonal psychotherapy for the nonpurging bulimic individual: A controlled comparison. *Journal of Consulting and Clinical Psychology, 61,* 296–305.

Wilfley, D. E., MacKenzie, K. R., Welch, R. R., Ayres, V. E., & Weissman, M. M. (2000). *Interpersonal psychotherapy for group*. New York: Basic Books.

Wilfley, D. E., Welch, R. R., Stein, R. I., Spurrell, E. B., Cohen, L. R., Saelen, B. E., et al. (2002). A randomized comparison of group cognitive-behavioral therapy and group interpersonal psychotherapy for the treatment of overweight individuals with binge-eating disorder. *Archives of General Psychiatry, 59,* 713–721.

Williams, J. B. W. (1988). A structured interview guide for the Hamilton Depression Rating Scale. *Archives of General Psychiatry, 45,* 742–747.

Willis, S. L., & Nesselroade, C. S. (1990). Long-term effects of fluid ability training in old-old age. *Developmental Psychology, 26,* 905–910.

Wolfson, L., Miller, M., Houck, P., Ehrenpreis, L., Stack, J., Frank, E., et al. (1997). Foci of interpersonal psychotherapy (IPT) in depressed elders: Clinical and outcome correlates in a combined IPT/nortriptyline protocol. *Psychotherapy Research, 7,* 45–55.

Wolkenstein, B. H., & Sterman, L. (1998). Unmet needs of older women in a clinic population: The discovery of possible long-term sequelae of domestic violence. *Professional Psychology: Research and Practice, 4,* 341–348.

Yesavage, J. A., Brink, T. L., Rose, T. L., Lum, O., Huang, V., Adey, M., & Leirer, V. O. (1983). Development and validation of a geriatric depression screening scale: A preliminary report. *Journal of Psychiatry Research, 17,* 37–49.

Youssef, F. A. (1990). The impact of group reminiscence counseling on a depressed elderly population. *Nurse Practitioner, 15,* 32–38.

Zisook, S., & Shuchter, S. R. (1991). Depression through the first year after the death of a spouse. *American Journal of Psychiatry, 148,* 1346–1352.

Zweig, R. A., & Hinrichsen, G. A. (1993). Factors associated with suicide attempts by depressed older adults: A prospective study. *American Journal of Psychiatry, 150,* 1687–1692.

INDEX

Access to care
    barriers to mental health care, 39–40
    for persons with interpersonal deficits, 153–154
    supply of geropsychologists, 40–41
Activities of daily living, 11–12
Adaptation
    cognitive functioning in older adults, 16
    IPT conceptualization, 44–45
Adjustment disorder, 76, 130
Administration on Aging, 7
Aging. See Geropsychology; Older adults
AIDS/HIV, 9, 57, 75, 101–102, 103, 135
Alzheimer's disease, 15. See also Dementia
American Association for Retired Persons, 8
Anxiety disorders, 59
Arthritis, 11
Assessment
    cognitive functioning, 31–32
    depression, 28–32, 48, 75–76, 79–80
    health status, 30–31
    interpersonal deficits, 155–156
    interpersonal role disputes, 114–118
    obstacles to, 29, 30
    for pharmacotherapy, 78
    role transition stress, 136, 137–138
    social relationships, 79
    time allotment for, 188–189
Assisted living, 18

Baby boom generation, 9–10, 19
Beck Depression Inventory, 32
Behavior change techniques in IPT for depression, 53
Bibliotherapy, 36
Bipolar disorder, 57–58
Butler, Robert, 7

Cancer, 11
Caregiver stress, 19, 37–38, 66
    IPT case example, 139–145, 152
    role engulfment, 138–139
    role transition and, 134, 136
Caregiver symbiosis, 139
Case examples, xiii

Certification of IPT practitioners, 199–200
Chronic disease epidemiology, 11
Clarification
    depression treatment, 52–53
    in grief work, 96
Cognitive–behavioral therapy, 79–80, 196
    depression treatment, 35–36, 38, 44
Cognitive functioning
    adaptation in older adults, 16
    assessment, 31–32, 76
    capacity for clinical response, 197
    instrumental activities of daily living, 11
    maintaining focus in therapy, 187–188
    normal aging, 15–16
    outcome predictor in depression treatment, 68
    types of intelligence, 15–16
    See also Alzheimer's disease
Cohort-related issues
    clinical significance, 4
    cognitive functioning, 15
    depression risk, 21, 22–23
Communication analysis, depression treatment, 53
Comprehensive Guide to Interpersonal Psychotherapy, 46, 47, 74, 198
Continuum-of-care communities, 18
Contract, therapy, 53, 191, 193
Cost of care
    barriers to mental health services, 40
    concerns of older adults, 13–14
    depression assessment, 28
Countertransference, 38–39
Crystallized intelligence, 15–16

Decision analysis, 53
Dementia
    causes, 16
    prevalence, 16
    risk, 16
    role transition stress for caregiver, 139–145, 152
    See also Alzheimer's disease
Demographic patterns and trends, xi, 8–10
    suicide risk, 24

Depression during and after pregnancy, 57
Depression in adolescents, 57
Depression in older persons
    assessment, 28–32, 48, 75–76, 79–80
    diagnosis, 76–77
    disability status and, 25
    epidemiology, 22–23
    etiology, 45
    health status and, 23–24, 25, 31, 61–62
    IPT effectiveness, *xi–xii*, 69–74
    life stress and, 26
    minor depressive disorder, 23, 28
    model of depression, 45–46, 47, 63–65,
        184–185
    outcome predictors, 66–67
    pharmacotherapy, 197
    precipitants, 79
    presentation, 23–24
    protective factors, 26
    social relationships and, 26, 27–28, 45–
        46, 61–62, 63–65, 111. *See also* In-
        terpersonal deficits; Interpersonal
        role disputes
    subdysthymic, 72–73
    suicide and, 24–25
    treatment goals, 47, 184
    treatment options, 197
    vascular depression, 24
    vulnerability, 21, 22–23, 24, 25–27
    See also IPT treatment of depression;
        Treatment of depression
Developmental models, 62–65
Diabetes, 11
Directive techniques, 53
Divorce, 18–19, 114
Doctor–patient relationship, 29
Double depression, 76
Dysthymia
    double depression, 76
    IPT for, 57

Electroconvulsive therapy, 33, 35
Emotional functioning
    encouragement of affect in depression
        treatment, 52
    expressed emotion and depression, 45,
        66–67
    therapeutic strategies for role transition
        stress, 137, 138
    See also Grief
Empirically supported treatment, *xi*, 38
    rationale, 46

Empowerment, 8
Empty-nest syndrome, 134
Environmental docility hypothesis, 64
Erikson, E., 62
Exploration
    depression treatment, 52
    grief treatment, 96–98
    of options for resolving interpersonal
        disputes, 116–117
Expressed emotion, depression and, 45, 66–
    67

Family relations, 18
    caregiving stress, 66
    depression and, 45, 66
    future prospects, 19
    parent–child conflict, 112, 114–115
Family role in treatment
    clinical assessment and, 30
    depression therapy for caregivers, 37–
        38
Fertility rates, 9
Financial issues, 12–15
    housing, 18
    income sources, 12–13
    suicide rate and, 24
    See also Cost of care
Fluid intelligence, 15–16
Foster care, 18
Freud, S., 62

Gay and lesbian couples, 112
Gender differences
    demographic patterns, 10
    economic status, 12
    grief and bereavement, 94
    health risks, 11
    life expectancy, 9
    residential patterns, 17
    suicide risk, 24
    widows and widowers, 17, 93
Generational equity, 8
Geriatric Depression Scale, 32
Geropsychology
    aging-related problems, 4–5
    cohort-related problems, 4
    future needs, 10
    scope of, 3
    supply of practitioners, 40–41
    therapist preparation, 198–199
Grief
    clinical features, 93–94

course of bereavement, 93
depression symptoms and, 95–96
interpersonal role disputes and, 109
IPT case examples, 81–84, 98–109
IPT treatment of, 47, 51, 63, 94–95, 192
outcome predictors, 94
selection of therapy focus, 190
social relationships in recovery from, 98
therapeutic strategies, 95–98
treatment goals, 95
Group therapy, 59

Hamilton Rating Scale for Depression, 32
Health care
barriers to mental health services, 39–
40
concerns of older adults, 13–14
See also Medicare
Health of older persons, 8
caregiver stress, 19
depression and, 23–24, 25, 31, 61–62
epidemiologic patterns, 11–12
housing issues and, 16–17
intake assessment, 30–31
marital relationship and, 19, 61–62
role transition stress, 133, 134–136
Heart disease, 11
Housing
home ownership, 12, 13
living with children, 17
quality of life and, 16–17
trends and patterns, 17–18
Hypertension, 11

Individual differences, 7, 10–11
cognitive functioning, 16
Instrumental activities of daily living, 11–12
International Society for Interpersonal Psychotherapy, 199
Interpersonal counseling, 57, 72–73
Interpersonal deficits, 47, 63–64
acute depression intervention, 154
barriers to care for persons with, 153–
154
IPT case examples, 89–91, 157–173
psychological effects, 153, 173–174
therapeutic relationship with client
with, 156–157, 165, 173, 174
treatment goals, 47, 80, 154–155
treatment strategies, 155–157
Interpersonal psychotherapy (IPT)
commonalities with other therapies, 196

conceptual basis, 44–45
cultural adaptation of, 196–197
distinguishing features, 47–48, 195–196
indications, 56–59
maintenance, 175–176, 179–180, 182
origins and development, 43–44
potential obstacles to success, 183–193
structure, 46
therapist preparation, 183–184, 198–
200
See also IPT treatment of depression;
Termination of therapy
Interpersonal Psychotherapy of Depression, 46
Interpersonal role disputes, 47
assessing prospects for resolution, 117
client motivation for resolving, 131
conjoint therapy, 117
depression risk, 111
exploration of options in therapy, 116–
117
grief and, 109
IPT case examples, 81–86, 118–131
parallel relationships, 117–118
participation of other party to the dispute, 192
perpetuation of, 118
psychiatric complications, 112
relationship termination as solution to,
115
role expectations, 115–116, 124
role-playing to explore, 117
sources of, 111–112
staging, 114–115
treatment goals, 51, 80, 112–113
treatment strategies, 51, 113–118
values conflict in, 116
IPT. *See* Interpersonal psychotherapy
IPT treatment of depression, 35
acute intervention, 47, 54–55
assessment, 75–76, 79–80, 188–189
case examples, 81–91
client attendance problems, 188
client capacity for change, 185
client feelings of hopelessness in, 188
client selection, 186–187
client understanding of depression, 76–
78, 83, 84, 89
client understanding of treatment, 80–
81, 83–84
clinician preparation for, 68
effectiveness, *xi–xii*, 38, 54–59, 67–74,
198

goals, 47, 48, 51, 80, 184
grief focus. *See* Grief
identification of therapy focus, 189–191
initial sessions, 48, 75–91, 188–191
intermediate sessions, 47, 51–52, 191–192
interpersonal deficits as focus of. *See* Interpersonal deficits
interpersonal role disputes as focus of. *See* Interpersonal role disputes
maintaining problem focus in, 187–188
maintenance treatment, 55–56, 57, 70–71, 179–180, 182, 193
model of depression, 45–46, 47, 63–65, 184–185, 196
with older adult, 46–47, 65–74
outcome predictors, 66–67
role transitions as focus of. *See* Role transitions
structure, 46–47, 48, 81
techniques, 52–53
therapeutic relationship in, 53–54
therapist adherence to IPT outline, 185–186
therapist leadership in, 186
See also Termination of therapy
IQ, 15

Klerman, Gerald, 43, 44

Levinson, 63
Life expectancy, 10
trends, 9
Life review therapy, 35, 37
Life stress
depression in older persons and, 26, 45
environmental docility hypothesis, 64
in role transitions, 133–134

Maintenance IPT, 55–56, 57, 70–71, 175–176
indications, 179–180, 182, 193
treatment strategies, 180
Marital relationship
caregiver stress in, 134, 136
conflict avoidance, 112
depression and, 27, 45
health status and, 19, 61–62
long-standing unhappy marriages, 114
quality, 19
sources of conflict, 111–112
spouse abuse, 130–131

See also Interpersonal role disputes
Marital status, 17, 18–19
suicide risk and, 24
See also Marital relationship
Medicaid, 13, 40
long-term care and, 14
Medicare, 12, 31
concerns about, 13
mental health care, 40
See also Medicare
Memory, aging effects, 16
Mini-Mental State Examination, 31–32
Monoamine oxidase inhibitors, 35

Naturally occurring retirement communities, 17
Net worth, 12, 13
Nortriptyline, 34, 69–70, 71–72
Nursing homes
challenges for clients with interpersonal deficits in, 173–174
costs, 14
patterns and trends, 17
service delivery in, 17–18

Older adults
capacity for change, 185
cognitive functioning, 15–16
definition and clinical conceptualization, 6, 7–8
demographic patterns and trends, *xi*, 8–10
developmental models, 62–63
empowerment, 8
financial issues, 12–15
health issues, 8, 11–12
individual differences, 7, 10–11
physical appearance, 12
psychotherapy effectiveness, *xi*
public perceptions, 6, 7, 8, 9
residential arrangements, 16–17
self-perception, 6–7
social role transitions, 61
social service programs and agencies, 7–8
See also Depression in older persons
Older Americans Act, 7
Outpatient care, 39

Personality traits
depression risk, 47
depression treatment goals, 47

Pharmacotherapy for depression, 33–35, 197
    assessment for, 78
    clinical evolution, 44
Piaget, J., 62
Posttraumatic stress disorder, 59
Poverty, 12
Pregnancy, depression treatment in, 57
Prescription drugs
    cost concerns, 13
    intake assessment, 31
    See also Pharmacotherapy for depression
Problem-solving therapy, 35, 36–37
Psychodynamic psychotherapy, 44, 196
    depression treatment, 35, 36
Public opinion and understanding
    aging trends, 9
    doctor–patient relationship, 29
    perceptions of aging, 6, 7, 8

Race/ethnicity
    clinical significance, 4, 10–11
    depression risk, 26
    distribution among older population, 10
    economic status, 12, 13
    health risks, 11
    suicide risk, 24
Reminiscence therapy, 36–37
Respiratory disease, 11
Retirement, 134
Role playing
    in exploration of interpersonal disputes,
        117
    in IPT for depression, 53
Role transitions, 47
    health-related, 133, 134–136
    IPT case examples, 86–88, 139–152
    managing release of affect in therapy,
        138
    self esteem and, 135–136
    social support during, 138–139
    as source of stress, 133–134, 152
    treatment goals, 51, 80, 134–136
    treatment strategies, 51–52, 136–139
    See also Social roles

Selective serotonin reuptake inhibitors, 34, 197
Self concept
    client understanding of depression, 77–
        78
    developmental models, 62–63
    health status, 11
    of older adults, 6–7

response to loss, 94
    See also Role transitions
Social relationships, 18
    assessment, 48, 79, 155–156
    depression risk and, 26, 27–28, 45–46,
        63–65
    in grief recovery, 98
    IPT for depression, 47, 51, 62
    nonmarital dyads, 112
    repetitive patterns, 117–118, 156, 174
    role transition support, 138–139
    See also Interpersonal deficits; Social
        roles
Social rhythm therapy, 57–58
Social roles, 16
    aging and, 61
    interpersonal role disputes, 47, 51, 80,
        81–86
    IPT for depression, 47
    See also Interpersonal role disputes; Role
        transitions
Social Security, 6, 10
    benefit structure, 14
    purpose, 14
    reliance on, 12, 13
    viability concerns, 14–15
Social services, 12
    eligibility, 7
    future needs, 10
    historical development, 7–8
    housing programs, 17
Sociocultural factors
    clinical significance, 4, 10–11
    depression risk, 21
Stereotypes, 6, 7
Stigmatization, 6
Stroke, 11
Substance use disorder treatment, 59
Suicidal behavior and ideation
    depression and, 24
    methods of suicide, 25
    risk factors, 66
    suicide rate, 24
    trends, 24
Sullivan, Harry Stack, 44–45
Supervision, 198–200

Termination of therapy, 52, 165, 171–172
    case examples, 181–182
    grieving in, 176–177
    indications for continuing therapy, 175–
        176, 179–180

with nonresponding client, 178–179
potential problems in, 192–193
prior discussion with client, 175, 176
review of client progress in, 177–178
therapeutic relationship and, 176, 181
Therapeutic relationship
client reliance on therapist, 165
with client with interpersonal deficits,
156–157, 173, 174
depression treatment, 53–54
establishing, 75
termination of therapy and, 176, 181
therapist attitudes toward aging, 38–39
Time-limited psychotherapy, 44, 182
Transference, 53, 173, 176
Treatment of depression
barriers to care, 39–40
in caregivers, 37–38
conceptual and technical development,
44

effectiveness, 33, 35, 36, 38, 54–59
electroconvulsive therapy, 33, 35
patient attitudes toward, 29
pharmacotherapy, 33–35, 44
psychotherapy, 33–34, 35–39, 44
resource assessment, 8
role of family in, 30
therapist factors, 38–39
treatment options, 33–34
See also IPT treatment of depression
Tricyclic antidepressants, 34

Vascular depression, 24
Veterans Affairs, Department of, 10

Weissman, Myrna, 43–44
Widows and widowers, 17, 93

ABOUT THE AUTHORS

Gregory A. Hinrichsen, PhD, is director of psychology training at The Zucker Hillside Hospital, North Shore–Long Island Jewish Health System, and associate professor of psychiatry at the Albert Einstein College of Medicine. During 30 years in the field of aging, he has provided clinical services, conducted research, directed psychology internship and fellowship programs, and held leadership roles in state and professional organizations. He is past president of the American Psychological Association's (APA) Division 12, Section II (Clinical Geropsychology) and past chair of APA's Committee on Aging. His research has addressed family issues in late-life depression, dementia, and first-episode schizophrenia; adaptation to medical problems; and geropsychological education. Dr. Hinrichsen is a graduate of Harvard College and New York University. He lives in New York City.

Kathleen F. Clougherty, LCSW, is a senior interpersonal psychotherapy (IPT) trainer and supervisor for the New York State Psychiatric Institute, a clinical instructor in social work at the Yale Child Study Center, Yale School of Medicine, and a private practitioner specializing in the treatment of depression in adolescents and adults. Ms. Clougherty has been a therapist and supervisor in several major IPT studies, including IPT with HIV-positive men and women with depression, people with dysthymia, and adolescents with depression in school-based mental health clinics. She was a codeveloper and cotrainer of an adaptation of group IPT in the first randomized psychotherapy trial in Africa. Ms. Clougherty has done extensive training and supervision, both nationally and internationally, for psychiatrists, psychologists, and social workers. She was trained in IPT by Dr. Gerald Klerman. Ms. Clougherty resides with her family in New York City and Montague, Massachusetts.